POCKET GUIDE TO
HATHA YOGA

MICHELE PICOZZI

THE CROSSING PRESS
FREEDOM, CALIFORNIA

My appreciation for assistance in preparing this book goes to the always helpful and generous librarians at the Rockrimmon branch of the Pikes Peak Library District, with special thanks to my loving and patient husband.

For information on bulk purchases or group discounts for this and other Crossing Press titles, please contact our Special Sales Manager at 800-777-1048 x214.

Visit our Web site on the Internet: www.crossingpress.com

Disclaimer:
Consult your health care provider on the suitability of these exercises given your particular health status. All the exercises in this book should be performed with care, and are undertaken at the reader's sole discretion and risk. The author and publisher expressly disclaim any and all liabilities and/or injuries resulting from the exercises included in this book.

Library of Congress Cataloging-in-Publication Data

Picozzi, Michele.
    Pocket guide to hatha yoga / Michele Picozzi.
        p. cm.
    ISBN 0-89594-911-3
    1. Yoga, Hatha. I. Title.
RA781.7.P53   1998
613.7'046--dc21

98-5022
CIP

Dedicated to all my yoga teachers, especially Marge Mc Clenon and Carl Dawson for their kindness, clarity, and devotion to the practice of hatha yoga and to their students.

Contents

What Is Hatha Yoga? 9

History of Yoga 18

How Hatha Yoga Is Practiced in the West 29

Starting a Hatha Yoga Practice .39

Basic Postures for Health and Relaxation 58

Pranayama: Working with the Breath 77

Meditation 86

Traditional Yogic Diet Principles 92

Appendix 99

Glossary 108

Resources 110

Preface

Yoga is meditation in motion. While yoga assumes different forms, hatha yoga has come to the forefront as an increasingly popular form of exercise in the United States. Complementing the physical form of yoga are *pranayama*, or conscious breathing, and meditation.

As a form of exercise, hatha yoga consists of *asanas*, or postures, that embody controlled movement, concentration, flexibility, and conscious breathing. About half of the nearly 200 asanas are practiced widely in the West. The postures range from the basic to the complex, from the easily accomplished to the very challenging. While the movements tend to be slow and controlled, they provide an invigorating workout for the mind and body, including the internal organs.

This guide provides basic yet educated information about yoga, focusing on hatha yoga. It serves as both a roadmap for the beginner and a comprehensive resource for the continuing student. With this book as a foundation, you will be well prepared to begin a serious practice, aided either by a qualified hatha yoga instructor or the many video and book resources available. *Namasté*.

What Is Hatha Yoga?

Yoga is skill in action.

—Bhagavad Gita

OVERVIEW

Yoga is one of India's six great ancient philosophies. A systematized body of knowledge, it represents the world's oldest method for spiritual and physical development. Modern scholars have further defined yoga as the classical Indian science that concerns itself with the search for the soul and the union between the individual, whose existence is finite, and the Divine, which is infinite.

Like any science, yoga is based on certain basic principles founded on logical conclusions and rational reasoning. The science of yoga is unique because it encompasses all the types of problems associated with the human condition. No other science can match the quality, content, methodical process, and contributions of yoga.

Noted yoga scholar, author, and historian Georg Feuerstein, Ph.D., says that yoga seeks to foster wholeness. The word *yoga* comes from the Sanskrit word *yuj* meaning "yoke" or "union." As a word, the meaning of *hatha* can best be understood by looking at its two component syllables: *ha* means "sun" and *tha* means "moon." Yoga is the union between them, suggesting that the healthy joining of opposites—in this case, the mind and body—leads to strength, vitality, and peace of mind.

TYPES OF YOGA

While hatha yoga is the most familiar kind practiced in the West, there are five other distinct and individual practices for the purpose of unifying both body and mind.

Hatha Yoga

Called the "forceful path," this is the yoga of physical well-being. In the modern Western approach, hatha yoga is used primarily as a form of physical therapy. It consists of *asana* (postures), *pranayama* (breathing exercises), *pratyahara* (nerve control), *dharma* (mind control), *dhyana* (meditation and spiritual enlightenment). Practice is preceded by the *yama-niyama*, the ten rules of the yoga code of morality.

Raja Yoga

Called the "royal path," raja yoga is commonly presented as an approach for cultivating the mind's potential for concentration and meditation or transcending the mind for the purpose of physical and mental discipline. Also known as "classical" yoga, it consists of eight "limbs":

1. moral discipline
2. self-restraint
3. posture
4. breath control
5. sensory inhibition
6. concentration
7. meditation
8. ecstasy

These components are found in many other branches of yoga as well. The practice of raja yoga typically starts with hatha yoga, which gives the body the needed health and strength to endure the hardships of more advanced stages of training.

Karma Yoga

Karma yoga is known as "enlightenment through work or action." It aims to lessen our natural tendencies to desire, which lead to actions that obscure our true identity. Karma yoga seeks to guide us to spiritual freedom through the discipline of work that is selfless and performed as a service to others.

Bhakti Yoga

Bhakti yoga seeks to cultivate an open heart and create a path for enlightenment through selfless love and devotion to the Divine, which is seen as being present in every person and thing.

Jnana yoga

This is the path of discernment and wisdom, as taught in the *Upanishads*, the ancient Hindu mystical texts, which teach distinguishing the real from the unreal, or true happiness from fleeting pleasure.

Tantra Yoga

Tantra yoga represents the path of self-transcendence through ritual means, including consecrated sexuality. It teaches that there is no gap between the Divine and the world and the Divine can be found in ordinary existence.

WHAT IS HATHA YOGA?

Often associated with Hinduism, yoga actually is older. It is thought to have evolved in the eleventh century as a way to prepare novices by giving them strength and equilibrium to meditate for long periods, as well as to serve as a beacon in a time the Hindus have called the *kali-yuga*, or the Dark

Ages of spiritual decline. Despite its long and deep connections to the past, hatha yoga is tailor-made for modern Westerners, as it is a holistic form of exercise. Indra Devi, one of hatha yoga's most respected modern teachers, calls yoga a science that gives a human being the knowledge of his or her true Self.

Hatha yoga, which means "yoga for health," symbolizes the physical aspect of the practice called yoga. It aims to balance different energy flows within the human body. Over the years, yoga has been met with misunderstanding, suspicion, and sometimes ridicule. However, these attitudes have changed gradually during the past thirty years, as more people take up yoga to increase flexibility and calm the mind. According to a recent Roper poll, six million Americans now practice hatha yoga. More recently, yoga's visibility and viability as an effective exercise program has been increased by the endorsements of celebrities such as Jane Fonda, Demi Moore, Woody Harrelson, and Sting.

Many people initially are attracted to hatha yoga for its ability to relieve the effects of stress, but it offers much more. Western doctors and scientists are discovering the health benefits of hatha yoga. Studies conducted abroad have shown that hatha yoga can relieve the symptoms of several common and potentially life-threatening illnesses, such as arthritis, arteriosclerosis, chronic fatigue, diabetes, AIDS, asthma, and obesity. Many believe it even fends off the ravages of old age.

A near-perfect fitness routine, hatha yoga provides the means for people of any age not only to get and stay in shape, but also to develop balance, coordination, and a sense of centeredness. It renews, invigorates, and heals the body—stretching and toning the muscles, joints, and spine and directing blood and oxygen to the internal organs (including the glands and nerves). Yoga is distinctly different from other kinds of exercise. It generates motion without causing strain and imbalances in the body. When practiced correctly, hatha yoga has no such negative effect on either the inner or outer body. No other form of exercise in existence today can make such a claim.

When done with dedication and purpose, hatha yoga can be a quite demanding, yet immensely rewarding type of exercise. While not inherently aerobic, it involves almost every muscle in the body and challenges the body to work in a different and often more passive way. Since the limbs function as free weights, resistance is created by moving the body's center of gravity. This strengthening gives way endurance as poses are held for longer periods of time.

Unlike conventional forms of exercise, such as weight training, walking, biking, or hiking, hatha yoga stresses quality of movement over quantity. A consistent hatha yoga practice can quiet the mind and refresh the body, bringing health, relaxation, and happiness. However, to reap the maximum benefits hatha yoga has to offer, the practice must be tailored to the needs and goals of the individual.

YOGA AND RELIGION

Yoga does not meet the traditional definitions of a religion. Rather than broadcasting a philosophy or doctrine of its own, hatha yoga is a physical and psychological discipline that combines the learning and practice of *asana*, *pranayama*, and meditation.

Because of its roots in Eastern religion and mythology, hatha yoga has often been associated with the Hindu religion. While both Hinduism and yoga have their roots in

India, yoga is an independent tradition. Its separate physical and psychological processes have no connection with religious beliefs. While yoga encourages vegetarianism and celibacy, these practices are not required to reap the many benefits hatha yoga has to offer.

There are, however, a set of ethics associated with yoga, which complements the practice of hatha yoga. While adherence to these ethics is not required, there is substantial benefit to be gained when followed. Additionally, dedicated hatha yoga practice has been found to enhance the religious practice or beliefs of practitioners, whatever their current beliefs.

COMPONENTS OF HATHA YOGA

Hatha yoga consists of three essential components.

Asana: derived from the Sanskrit root meaning "to stay," "to be," "to sit," or "to be established in a particular position". The word refers specifically to all yoga postures or exercises that encourage flexibility and strengthen the skeletal, muscular, glandular, and nervous systems. The spine functions as the focal point of many of the postures, and all postures require a conscious awareness, steadiness, and the ability to surrender to gravity. Patañjali, author of the bible of yoga, the *Yoga Sutras*, describes *asana* as the place on which the student sits or stands and that both the student and the posture are firm and relaxed.

Pranayama: concerns breathing practice where *prana*, vital air or energy, is contained and balanced; *yama* is the control and direction of that energy and is gained by conscious inhalation, breath retention, and exhalation. Regular practice regulates and harmonizes the breath and its rhythm. The compelling force behind relaxation in yoga comes from *pranayama*, or breath awareness, which increases mental and physical energy by releasing the mind from its continuous stream of random thoughts.

For thousands of years, Eastern medical practitioners have believed breathing to be the single most important factor in health, but only recently has the West caught on. Today, the combination of controlled breathing and meditation are at the core of well-known stress-reduction programs offered at the University of Massachusetts Medical Center in Worcester and the Menniger Clinic in Topeka, Kansas.

Meditation—*Pratyahara*—is withdrawal of the senses from the outer world. *Dharana* (concentration), *dhyana* (contemplation or absorption/meditation), and *samadhi* (ecstatic union) are the final stages of practice and are collectively known as meditation. Like the word *yoga*, meditation refers to the goal of ecstatic union and the variety of practices used to reach this goal. Meditation could be broadly defined as a focusing of attention that results in quieting the mind, increasing intuition, and the ability to relax at will.

SPECIFIC HEALTH BENEFITS

Yoga is both preventive and therapeutic. It is one of the very few exercises that invert the body, as in postures such as headstand, handstand, shoulderstand, and others. Regularly turning the body upside down defies gravity and brings blood to areas of the body that are starved for oxygen and nourishment.

Yoga postures stretch and relax muscles and properly align the body, thus giving overworked muscles a chance to rest. Through proper alignment, problems can be avoided before they start, and present imbalances caused by poor posture can be addressed.

Besides its ability to strengthen the body, hatha yoga also has a relaxation component, an aspect that many people find attractive. Muscles that are chronically tense and cause pain have the chance to loosen and lengthen, thus engendering relaxation. Yoga, while it doesn't work as quickly or conveniently as popping an aspirin or prescription anti-inflammatory, will uncover the underlying causes of chronic muscle tension and pain and lead to a more permanent and ultimately healthy resolution.

Yoga and the ancient Indian healing tradition of *ayurveda* are closely connected. *Ayurveda*, which means science of life, is based on wholeness—the idea that the body, mind, and spirit are one, each affecting the other. Both yoga and *ayurveda* support the mind-body connection to health and well-being.

Since it has profound physiological and psychological affects on the body, yoga is increasingly prescribed to counteract a variety of physical problems, addictions, and postural abnormalities.

Physical Benefits

Yoga has been shown to offer the following physical benefits to the body:

- promotes suppleness of spine and joints
- strengthens, tones, and builds muscles
- stimulates the glands of the endocrine system
- improves digestion and elimination
- increases circulation
- relaxes the nervous system
- boosts immune response
- refreshes the body by relieving muscle strain

- increases stamina
- decreases cholesterol and blood sugar levels
- invites balance and grace
- increases body awareness
- encourages weight loss

Mental Benefits

Because of its meditative aspects, both in practice of the postures and in single-pointed concentration in meditation, yoga functions as a mental discipline as well.

Yoga's ability to calm and quiet the mind has a physiological basis. Anxiety leads to a fight-or-flight response in the body, which leads to specific physiological responses, such as, the release of hormones, adrenaline in particular, that trigger shallow breathing, muscle tension, and rapid heartbeat. Yoga interrupts this mechanism by calming a busy or agitated mind, providing a stabilizing influence. Specific benefits include:

- quiets the mind
- centers attention
- sharpens concentration
- frees the spirit

History of Yoga

THE ESSENCE OF YOGA

As both science and art, yoga offers the necessary tools to live fully and consciously. The ancient yogic scriptures assert that no effort is lost on the yogic path, which truly is a lifelong endeavor. Dedicated practice of yoga goes beyond the boundaries of religion and surpasses the notion that to practice yoga means legs up, head down, and a few vegetables a day. Like anything of value, practicing hatha yoga is a process; it is about wholeness, integration, stillness, and interconnectedness.

In this hurried and often troubled world, yoga serves as a tremendous resource. While yoga is most often identified today as a stress reduction method, it does far more than lessen the tension and stiffness in our bodies. When practiced regularly, yoga can be a potent tool for healing and personal transformation, opening our hearts and minds to new ways of caring for others and empowering ourselves.

THE LANGUAGE OF YOGA

Sanskrit, the ancient Indian language, is the language of yoga. Literally translated, *Sanskrit* means mathematically and scientifically exact language. In it's written form, Sanskrit is perfectly phonetic. The Sanskrit alphabet consists of a logical array of vocal sounds, and each letter represents a basic root word. Since all Sanskrit words are built upon this guiding principle, it can be applied like a formula, making Sanskrit a relatively easy language to learn.

Historians have theorized that most Indo-Aryan languages, including English, have their origins in a language similar to Vedic Sanskrit. The first serious translations of yogic texts from Sanskrit to English in the West took place during the Victorian era.

The word *yoga* has its roots in the Sanskrit word *yuj*, meaning to merge, join, or unite. Classical yoga uses Sanskrit for the names of the *asanas* (poses or postures) and *pranayama* (breathing) techniques, and these names are still used throughout the world today. Becoming familiar with Sanskrit words as you practice yoga has some distinct advantages. Many styles of yoga, especially the Iyengar system of hatha yoga, refer to the *asanas* by their Sanskrit names, which describe the shape or function of the postures or reflect the names of ancient Indian gods and sages or animals and birds. Using the Sanskrit names provides a foundation for further exploration of yogic texts and philosophy and establishes a connection between the ancient art and modern practice of yoga.

THE DEVELOPMENT OF YOGA THROUGH THE AGES

Indian culture has always absorbed ideas and beliefs from many diverse sources. The history of yoga is intrinsically connected with the development of Hinduism and Buddhism. The exact origins of modern yoga are unknown, but it is thought to be about five thousand years old.

The earliest evidence of yoga practice can be traced to the highly-developed civilization that flourished in the Indus Valley thousands of years before Christ's birth. In the ancient cities of Mojendro-Daro in Northern India and Harappa (in what is now known as Pakistan), stone sculptures depict seated figures in yoga positions and in meditation. The first written reference to yoga came between 3000 B.C. and 1200 B.C., with the appearance of the *Vedas*, the central texts of Indian religion and mysticism and the culture's earliest known literature. The *Vedas* later became known as the *Upanishads*, which means "to sit next to" in Sanskrit. The *Upanishads* contain the first written reference to yoga and meditation in this passage: "When the five senses and the mind are still, and reason itself rests in silence, then begins the path supreme. This calm steadiness of the senses is called yoga."

YOGA SUTRAS

The most widely acknowledged text on the system of yoga is the *Yoga Sutras* (*sutras* means "threads" in Sanskrit). Basically, the *Yoga Sutras* consist of aphorisms to guide yoga practice. While ancient they remain widely read and followed today. The work is attributed to the physician, sage, and scholar Patañjali. Patañjali, who was the first person to put the verbal teachings of yoga into writings, is often referred to as the "father of yoga." He defines yoga as the "stilling of the restless mind."

The four volumes of proverbs that comprise the *Yoga Sutras* serve as a distillation of the essence of yoga teaching as it has been passed down orally from ancient times. They offer succinct, practical statements on how to concentrate the mind through correct practice. They also discuss the ethical precepts, or *yamas*, that govern social responsibilities and relationships with others, including nonviolence, and *niyamas*, which represent the fundamentals of all yoga practice. At the core of these systematic teachings is what is known as the Eight-fold Path.

The Eight-fold Path

In second chapter of the *Yoga Sutras*, Patañjali describes the eight steps of classical yoga, often referred to as the

Eight-fold Path. These steps offer seekers the means and methods to still the mind.

Meant to complement each other, they are fundamental to practicing meditation, correct posture, and stable breathing.

The components of the Eight-fold Path include:

- *yama*—moral restraint
- *niyama*—personal discipline
- *asana*—posture
- *pranayama*—breath control
- *pratyahara*—control of the senses
- *dharana*—concentration
- *dhyana*—meditation
- *samadhi*—contemplation

Another classic Indian text, the epic poem *Bhagavad Gita*, written several hundred years later, describes yoga as the "path of the Eternal and freedom from bondage." The *Bhagavad Gita* remains in wide use in India as well as other parts of the world. It details the various meanings of yoga, some of which include:

- equilibrium in success and failure
- skill in action
- supreme secret of life
- producer of the greatest felicity, serenity, nonattachment
- destroyer of pain

In his search for enlightenment, Buddha practiced yoga, and the great Indian leader Ghandi was said to have gleaned solace and resolution from yoga.

Descriptions of the postures and breathing exercises that form the core of hatha yoga were written down beginning around A.D. 1000. These writings emphasized not only the health and longevity the postures would bring to devoted practitioners, but also the significance of meditation and moral discipline.

Traditionally, disciples were men who turned to yoga in their later years, when their children were grown and their responsibilities as householders had been fulfilled. They studied under the direct supervision of a *guru*, or teacher, who was viewed as the embodiment of the Divine. Surrender to the guru was absolute, and his authority was not questioned. The guru-disciple relationship assumed that the aspirant was ready for the renunciation and devotion that total commitment to the spiritual life required, and the guru rejected students deemed not ready for rigors of study.

The British colonization of India introduced yoga to the West, as the British governor-general encouraged the study of Sanskrit. Subsequently, translations of the *Bhagavad Gita* and the *Sacred Books of the East* from Sanskrit into English did much to spread Indian philosophy.

HOW YOGA CAME TO AMERICA

Hatha yoga made its debut in the United States in the mid-1800s among groups of intellectual writers interested in the esoteric philosophies of the East. These literary lions included the likes of Ralph Waldo Emerson, Henry David Thoreau, and Bronson Alcott. Later, a slim volume entitled *Light in Asia*, a Victorian–era biography of Gautama Buddha, sold half a million copies, and as a result, societies promoting Eastern thought emerged.

One of the featured attractions of the 1893 Chicago World's Fair was the appearance of Swami Vivekananda (1863-1902), one of India's most celebrated sages. While in America, he taught raja yoga; he also spent two years teaching in Detroit, Chicago, Boston, New York, and Europe. His presence was credited with further stimulating the West's interest in yoga, which opened the door for other teachers to come to this country.

Hollywood was introduced to the health benefits of hatha yoga in the 1940s, when the Russian-born yoga teacher Indra Devi migrated there. Twenty years later, the combination of the cultural changes initiated in the 1960s, including the growing interest in Eastern religions and the publication of Jess Stearn's best-seller *Yoga, Youth & Reincarnation* (Bantam Books) in 1965 caused yoga to permeate more and more of American culture.

FAMOUS HATHA YOGA TEACHERS
Krishnamacharya

This long-lived teacher (1888-1989) may well be the father of modern hatha yoga, for he was the teacher of such subsequent influential teachers as K. Pattabhi Jobs, who is credited with developing ashtanga yoga; B. K. S. Iyengar; and Indra Devi. His son Desikachar (and nephew of B. K. S. Iyengar) is a yoga master in his own right. All of his students went on to carry his teaching to the West, mostly in the United States, Canada, and Europe. He is credited with advancing at least four major branches of hatha yoga in the United States alone.

From 1930 to 1950, he served as the head of the Yoga Institute at the royal palace of Mysore. While there, he presided over the palace's yoga academy, where he gained a reputation as a yoga therapist, helping people with a variety of physical ailments. Revered as a prolific sage, Krishnamacharya authored dozens of books on yoga.

T. K. V. Desikachar

After receiving a Western education and degree in structural engineering, the son of the late, great yoga master Krishnamacharya and nephew of B. K. S. Iyengar returned to India in the 1960s to teach yoga. His style of hatha yoga, is based on the principle of *vinyasa krama*, which translates as "an intelligently conceived step-by-step-approach to the teaching of *asana*."

He teaches at the school named in honor of his father, the Krishnamacharya Yoga Mandiram in Madras, India. He has been a pioneer in researching yoga's positive effect on cases of schizophrenia, depression, mental retardation, asthma, and diabetes.

B. K. S. Iyengar

B. K. S. Iyengar is considered by many to be one of the world's foremost proponents of hatha yoga living today. Many prominent world figures, including the acclaimed violinist Yehudi Menuhin and Queen Beatrice of Holland, and thousands of ordinary people practice Iyengar-style hatha yoga.

Iyengar is credited with developing the therapeutic side of hatha yoga, based on anatomical principles. He was the first to introduce props to accommodate students with physical limitations. He is also the author of the timeless work *Light on Yoga* (Schocken Books, 1979), a comprehensive review of 200 *asanas* with instruction in the basics of yoga philosophy and *pranayama*, as well as *Light on Pranayama* (The Crossroad Publishing Company, 1987), *Light on the Yoga Sutras of Patañjali* (Thorsons Publishing, 1993), and *The Tree of Yoga* (Fine Line Books, 1988).

Known for his strict teaching techniques and dynamic personality, he has been called the "Lion of Pune." In 1974, he founded the Ramamani Iyengar Memorial Yoga Institute in Pune, India, named in honor of his late wife, and made his inaugural visit to the United States. Both his children—daughter Geeta, author of *Yoga: A Gem for Women* (Timeless Books, 1990), and son Prashant, a yogic scholar—teach at the institute.

K. Patahbi Jois

A disciple of Krishnamacharya, Jois is credited with developing the physically challenging style of hatha yoga known as ashtanga, based on six prescribed sequences of postures for the purpose of heating and thus detoxifying the body. This style is different from the ashtanga yoga, or Eight-fold Path of Patañjali. Jois is the founder of the Ashtanga Yoga Institute located in Mysore, India.

Yogi Bhajan

A Sikh, Bhajan brought the secrets of Kundalini yoga to the West in 1969. He went on to found the 3HO Foundation (for happy, healthy, holy), which maintains headquarters in Los Angeles and New Mexico.

Yogi Amrit Desai

Originally an Indian master of Kundalini, Desai is credited with developing Kripalu yoga.

Paramhansa Yogananda

One of the earliest yogic masters to bring yoga to the West, Yogananda (1893-1952) is the author of the world-famous book *Autobiography of a Yogi* (Self-Realization Fellowship, 1946) and founder of the Self-Realization Fellowship. His book, now more than a half century old, is responsible for introducing thousands to meditation and hatha yoga.

Swami Kriyananda

Born James Donald Walters, Kriyananda was a disciple of Paramhansa Yogananda and also publicly practiced kriya yoga. Kriyananda went on to establish the Ananda World Brotherhood Village, a residential community located in Nevada City, California.

Swami Sivananda

A sage from Rishikesh, India, Sivananda wrote dozens of books on the different aspects of yoga. He is credited with furthering the development of hatha yoga taught in the United States. His disciples included Swami Satchidananda and Swami Vishu-devananda.

Indra Devi

Born Eugenie Peterson in 1899 in Russia, Devi's interest in yoga started at an early age. After studying drama in Germany, she moved to India in 1930 to study yoga. There she studied with Krishnamacharya and Swami Somnathasbram and acted in Indian films under the name Indra Devi.

In 1947, she moved to the United States, where she introduced yoga to Hollywood. Her famous pupils included actors Robert Ryan, Jennifer Jones, Greta Garbo, and Gloria Swanson. Ten years later, Devi officially became a U.S. citizen, and two years later she published *Yoga for Americans*. She has taught yoga for more than seventy years in such diverse locations as India, China, Argentina, and Mexico.

Richard Hittleman

Hittleman (1927-1991) took his first yoga class in 1936 from a Hindi handyman who worked on the family estate located in upstate New York. He began teaching yoga in the late 1940s, while studying for a master's degree at Columbia University Teacher's College. Realizing yoga would appear exotic to 1950s America, he stressed yoga's benefits of physical well-being, such as stress reduction, stamina, coordination, weight regulation, firming the muscles, and quieting the mind. Many credit him with leading the hatha yoga boom of the 1970s with his nationally televised television program, which began airing from Los Angeles in 1961.

Lilias Folan

Following on the heels of Hittleman's successful TV yoga classes, Folan, who became a student of yoga in 1964 and studied with Indian masters in the United States, Canada, and India, launched the popular PBS series, *Lilias, Yoga & You* in 1970. By 1977, 200 stations carried the Cincinnati, Ohio-based program. *Time* magazine called her "the Julia Child of yoga."

Folan combines hatha yoga with the introspective aspects of yoga, especially *bhakti* yoga and *jnana* yoga. She is the author of *Lilias, Yoga and Your Life* (Macmillan, 1981) and several popular videos on learning and practicing hatha yoga.

Bikram Choudhury

Born in 1945, Choudhury is the youngest of the gurus from India who have influenced the growth of yoga in America. The system of yoga he developed was based on the teachings of Bishnu Ghosh, the brother of Paramhansa Yogananda. It consists of a twenty-six-posture sequence done in a pre-scribed order. Choudhury claims this practice allows students to attain "100 percent of a pure internal body."

He migrated in 1970 from Calcutta to the United States and opened the first of many Yoga Colleges of India. He eventually became known as "Yogi to the stars," having taught Raquel Welch and basketball star Kareem Abdul Jabar. He now oversees 150 branch centers in fifty countries.

Swami Satchidananda

Satchidananda is the author of *Integral Hatha Yoga*, considered the "bible of yoga" by Americans when it was introduced here in the 1970s. Before that, his claim to fame in the yoga world was introducing the masses attending Woodstock to the classic chant "*Om*."

Swami Vishu-devananda

Vishu-devananda is the author of the *Complete Illustrated Book of Yoga* (1960), which inspired Western students. His teachings promote the practice of yogic postures, breathing exercises, relaxation, a vegetarian diet, meditation, and positive thinking.

How Hatha Yoga Is Practiced in the West

YOGA TODAY

The more common stereotypical images of yoga—from turban-wearing swamis to snake charmers to people turning themselves into human pretzels or levitating—have gone the way of love beads and bell bottom pants. Hatha yoga, which emphasizes *asana* (practice of postures), *pranayama* (breathing techniques), and *dhyana* (meditation), is the most commonly practiced form of yoga in the West. Hatha yoga attracts people from all walks of life—children, senior citizens, women as well as men—and is readily accessible to people who aren't interested in advancing or developing a personal spiritual practice.

Different styles or forms of hatha yoga can be found in nearly every part of the United States. Many consider it as normal a form of exercise as walking or biking. It is taught everywhere, from TV to local YMCAs and YWCAs as well as at spas, gyms, community and senior centers, and private studios dedicated solely to teaching and practicing yoga.

Yoga also is increasingly embraced by the medical community. Popular health practitioners who possess mainstream medical credentials and are open to alternative practices include Andrew Weil, M.D., Dean Ornish, M.D., Joan Borysenko, M.D., and Jon Kabat-Zinn, Ph.D. Such practitioners have long encouraged patients and clients to take up yoga. Yoga is also an integral part of many stress management programs endorsed and paid for by HMOs and insurance companies. In fact, Cedars-Sinai Medical Center's Preventive and Rehabilitative Cardiac Center includes gentle yoga postures and breathing techniques to aid the recovery of patients with heart disease.

The most often cited reasons Westerners begin a yoga practice are to:

- increase flexibility
- promote relaxation
- manage stress
- complement a fitness program
- heal an injury or strengthen a weak back

HEALTH BENEFITS OF HATHA YOGA

Like other Eastern forms regarded as "movement arts," hatha yoga, particularly from a physical standpoint, offers both preventive and therapeutic aspects. A complete fitness program, hatha yoga will release endorphins in the brain as well as any regular exercise program. Yoga postures stretch, extend, and flex the spine, while exercising muscles and joints, keeping the body strong and supple. And when done in conjunction with breathing techniques, hatha yoga postures stimulate circulation, digestion, and the nervous and endocrine systems.

As a workout, yoga can be intense, easy, or somewhere in between. It can be practiced by anyone, regardless of age, to achieve a more limber body, increased physical coordination, better posture, and improved flexibility without incurring the potentially negative effects associated with high-impact forms of exercise.

Hatha yoga remains different from newer or more modern types of exercise. It does not aim to raise the heart rate (although variations such as Ashtanga, Power Yoga, or the flow series taught by Bikram Choudhury may) or work on specific muscle groups. Overall, the postures release stiffness and tension, help to reestablish the inner balance of the spine, renew energy, and restore health. Some postures provide the added benefit of being weight-bearing, which helps sustain bone mass (very important for women). Relaxation and breathing exercises produce stability and reduce stress and put you in touch with your inner strength. In addition, regular practice of hatha yoga can promote graceful aging. Famous yoga teachers Vanda Scavelli and Indra Devi, along with many not-so-famous people, maintain a daily yoga practice well into their eighties and nineties.

According to Mary Schatz, M.D., author of *Back Care Basics* (Rodmell Press, 1992), the psychological and physiological determinants of good health are indeed integral components of the ancient science of yoga. She writes: "Yoga provides the means to become physically fit in the context of a philosophy that encourages positive health practices and personality characteristics. The body is no longer divorced from the mind and the spirit. There is a clear correlation between yoga and the positive health practices documented in medical literature."

Some of the documented health benefits attributed to yoga include:

- relieves chronic stress patterns in the body
- lengthens, strengthens, and tones muscles
- corrects posture
- improves muscular-skeletal conditions such as bad knees, tight shoulders and neck, bunions, swayback, and scoliosis
- boosts immune function
- increases fitness levels and refines balance
- fosters healthy body awareness
- manages stress and hypertension
- improves concentration

One of the hidden benefits of studying and practicing hatha yoga is the ability to take care of yourself. If your back goes out or leg cramps keep you awake at night, a yoga posture or series of postures will help relieve the discomfort.

HATHA YOGA SYSTEMS

Because of hatha yoga's ever increasing popularity in the West, a wide variety of yoga styles have grown up around particular teachers from India or as variations on a theme developed by a Western teacher. Like individuals, styles or schools of hatha yoga have their own personalities and approaches to practicing *asanas*. What distinguishes the different styles is what's emphasized, be it posture, breath, aerobics, dance, slow and rhythmic movements, philosophy, or a combination of many factors.

Although the basic *asanas* and breathing exercises remain the same, how they are done, in what order, and where attention is focused while doing them constitute the main differences among the many schools. However, no matter which style you opt for, special clothing isn't required. All that's needed are comfortable, loose or stretchy clothes, bare feet, an empty stomach, open mind, and a few basic props.

Hatha Yoga Traditions Practiced and Taught in the West

Ananada Yoga

This method combines the physical and spiritual. Each pose is integrated with a specific affirmation to develop or heighten self-awareness. Ananada yoga also teaches a series of poses called "energization exercises." These exercises involve tensing and relaxing different parts of the body, coupled with breathing exercises to send energy to them. Deep relaxation in the poses as a preparation for meditation is also stressed. Classes and a one-month teacher training program are offered at the Expanding Light facility in Nevada City, California, as well as other cities in the western United States and in Assisi, Italy.

Ashtanga Yoga

Consisting of 240 postures done in six successive series (*vinyasa*) linked by the breath, Ashtanga yoga represents the most intensive form of hatha yoga, requiring great stamina and flexibility.

The concentrated sequencing of postures is designed to create *tapas*, or heat, inside the body for the purpose of cleansing and detoxifying the body to bring forth *prana*, or to breathe, so it can be channeled up through the spine. Ashtanga also emphasizes strength and flexibility.

Very few teachers are certified to teach Ashtanga yoga in the West. Contact the Ashtanga Yoga Center (see Resources) for more information.

Iyengar Yoga

Probably the most widely known style of hatha yoga in the West, this style of hatha yoga is based on the teachings of B. K. S. Iyengar. It is regarded mostly for its rigorous scientific and therapeutic approach, concentrating on correcting structural imbalances in the physical body.

The distinguishing characteristics of the Iyengar style include the extensive use of props—blankets, sticky mats, folding chairs, wood blocks and benches, bolsters, and straps—and attention to detail, from correct posture to the placement of hands, pelvis, and feet.

Classes typically focus in great detail on only a few *asanas* so as to refine movements. Beginning students are drilled in standing poses so as to learn proper alignment and balance, which is necessary in other poses. After a foundation has been established, students are then taught *pranayama*.

Teachers undergo a rigorous certification program and are taught anatomy, physiology and kinesiology as well as yoga philosophy. There are Iyengar institutes, centers, and independent teachers throughout the world, particularly in the United States and Europe.

Integral Yoga

Based on the teachings of Swami Satchindananda, Integral Yoga emphasizes a more meditative rather than anatomical approach. It combines all the paths of yoga—*asana*, *pranayama*, selfless service, prayer, chanting, meditation, and self-inquiry—into one approach.

Kripalu Yoga

Less concerned with the structural detail of the postures, Kripalu yoga has been described as "meditation in motion." It emphasizes the student's mental and emotional states as the poses are held, while encouraging a gentle, compassionate, and introspective approach. Postures are held for a long time so as to explore and release emotional and spiritual blocks.

This inner-directed form of hatha yoga consists of three stages: willful practice, will and surrender, and finally, surrendering to the body's wisdom. Within each of the three stages, poses are offered in different intensities: gentle, moderate, and vigorous. In addition, spontaneous postures and sequences of postures are encouraged, guided by the body's internal awareness.

The Kripalu Center for Yoga and Health, located in Lenox, Massachusetts, offers certificate programs in teacher training, workshops, retreats, and conferences.

Kundalini Yoga
Designed to bring forth the reservoir of energy (*kundalini*) stored at the base of the spine, this style of hatha yoga focuses on arousing the *kundalini* energy, using a combination of breath, posture, chanting, and meditation to direct this energy through the energy centers (*chakras*) located along the spine.

Several breathing techniques are highlighted including alternate nostril breathing, slow diaphragmatic breathing, and the "breath of fire".

Founder Yogi Bhajan's Healthy, Happy, Holy Organization (3HO) focuses on all aspects of the yogic lifestyle, as well as community service. There are approximately 1,500 Kundalini teachers, located primarily in the United States, Canada, Europe, Mexico, and South America.

Sivananda Yoga
Originated by Swami Vishnu-devananda, Sivananda Yoga is similar to Integral Yoga, with the same dietary restrictions and scriptural study.

Viniyoga
Originated by T. K. V. Desikachar, the style of hatha yoga called *viniyoga* is said to represent a middle path between the exactness of Iyengar yoga and physically demanding Ashtanga yoga. It is based on the principle of *vinyasa krama*, which means "an organized course of Yoga study," and combines *asana*, *pranayama*, meditation, text study,

counseling, imagery, prayer, chanting, and ritual.

Yoga postures are tailored to the physical needs and limitations of each student, taking into account body type, emotional needs, cultural heritage, and interest. Emphasis is on the spine, and breath is considered more important than how the posture is done. Typically, classes are private one-on-one sessions.

Yoga College of India

Classes consist of a two-part series of twenty-six repeating postures with two *pranayama* exercises that are designed to stretch and tone the whole body. Most poses are done twice and held for a minimum of ten seconds in a room with temperatures of eighty degrees or higher, often supplemented by moist air a humidifier. Class concludes with a brief period of relaxation.

Founded by Bikram Choudhury, the Yoga College of India has locations in Beverly Hills (classes and teacher training), San Francisco, Honolulu, and Tokyo. Classes are also taught at private studios throughout the United States.

Hatha Yoga Traditions Based on Eastern Philosophy and Developed by Westerners

Hidden Language Yoga

Developed by Swami Sivananda Radha, who was born Sylvia Hellman in 1911, this method of hatha yoga blends postures with journal writing and group discussion to investigate the symbolic meaning of each *asana* and the posture's effect on the student's mind and body.

Hidden Language Yoga borrows from Ananda yoga and Jungian theory while using symbol and metaphor to aid students in developing deeper awareness of the psychological and mystical messages of the poses. Swami Radha established the Yasodhara Ashram, an eighty-three-acre retreat at Kootenay Bay in British Columbia, Canada, and also is the founder of the Association for the Potential for Human Development in the United States.

Ishta Yoga
Originated by South African Mani Finger, Ishta yoga (Integral Sciences of Hatha and Tantric Arts) combines *asana* with *pranayama*, visualization, and guided meditation to open the body's subtle energy channels. Individual practice consists of a mantra with a set of postures tailored to the specific needs of the student. Finger's son Alan has been largely responsible for bringing Ishta yoga to the United States.

Jivamukti
Created in the early 1990s by New Yorkers Sharon Gannon and David Life, *Jivamukti* is a Sanskrit word that means "liberation while alive in the body." This system borrows from several styles of yoga, including Ashtanga, Iyengar, and Sivananda. Spiritual teachings are taught in tandem with postures. During class teachers chant in Sanskrit and read and interpret the philosophical teachings of yoga.

Phoenix Rising
Developed by Michael Lee in 1984, Phoenix Rising yoga therapy is based on Kripalu yoga. Lee intended it as a way for people to use yoga as a tool for living. It incorporates poses to support inner awareness, mental clarity, emotional stability, spiritual attunement, and physical well-being. It features sixteen basic poses, including forward bends

and backbends, inversions, and twisting poses. Phoenix Rising is done with a therapist, who gently holds the student until emotional tensions begin to surface and release, followed by a one-to-one discussion and concluded with a guided meditation.

Tri Yoga

Tri Yoga refers to the union of *asana*, *mudra* (practices similiar to *asanas*), and *pranayama*. Kali Ray of Aptos, California, founded Tri Yoga, which employs three designated practices that range from basic to advanced levels with other sequences tailored to a student's individual needs. Ray is also the creator of the Devi Dance, a performance that delivers yoga, *pranayama*, and meditation accompanied by music and done in flowing sequence.

Classes consist of a spontaneous, dance-like series of poses taught at a varied pace and accompanied by background music. Sessions are completed with seated *pranayama* and meditation.

White Lotus Yoga

Developed by Ganga White and Tracey Rich, this style represents a modified version of the Ashtanga style of hatha yoga. Characterized by a flowing style of practice, postures are done in flowing sequences that are characterized as lengthy and even aerobic. Classes are taught in Los Angeles at the Center for Yoga and at White Lotus Foundation's retreat center in Santa Barbara, California, where White has been director since 1973.

Starting a
Hatha Yoga Practice

Anybody who wants to can practice yoga. Anybody who can breathe; therefore anybody can practice yoga.

—T. K. V. Desikachar

HOW TO MAKE YOGA WORK FOR YOU

Hatha yoga has stood the test of time. It is the oldest physical discipline in existence, having been practiced for thousands of years. The original purpose of the postures and breathing exercises was to bring stability and relaxation so practitioners could prepare for the rigors of meditation, sitting still and alert for long periods of time.

Whether or not there is a clear goal in mind at the start (losing weight, relieving stress, practicing relaxation, gaining flexibility, strengthening the lower back, gaining peace of mind, enhancing overall physical well–being) dedicated, observant practice will help develop the capacity to set and achieve your goals. By its very nature, hatha yoga brings into balance the dissimilar aspects of the mind, body, and personality.

When planning to start a hatha yoga practice, you need to consider current abilities and physical limitations, as well as what you want to accomplish. Before beginning, the *Yoga Sutras* advise *vinyasa krama* (to place in a special way). One of the foremost teachers of hatha yoga, T. K. V. Desikachar explains the concept this way: "It is not enough to simply take a step as that step needs to take us in the right direction and be made in the right way...thus *vinyasa krama* describes a correctly organized course of yoga practice."

Ideally, your yoga practice should initially be focused on learning and becoming grounded in the basics of hatha yoga and its *asanas*. With this background, you can then center your yoga sessions around the demands of your lifestyle. If your work keeps you in front of a computer, or if you are on your feet a lot, the poses you will want to concentrate on will be different from those for someone who is preparing to run marathons or someone who has a chronic heart condition. Different people require different styles and different practices.

FINDING THE STYLE THAT'S RIGHT FOR YOU

Each of us comes to yoga in our own time and in our own way, much as the old proverb describes it: When the student is ready, the teacher appears. To decide on which kind of hatha yoga is right for you, you need to take into account your own personality and goals. The therapeutic aspect of yoga may be important if you are recovering from a sports injury or if chronic back pain plagues you, or the more cerebral or meditative aspects of yoga may be more appealing. If you aren't sure what you want to obtain from practicing yoga, sample classes of different styles of hatha yoga from different teachers. If a variety of styles or teachers isn't available, check your local library for videotapes to preview at your own pace and at little cost.

As there are widely differing techniques and styles of practice and sometimes conflicting points of view, you will want to take the time to find the methods and teacher that are right for you and to assess intelligently and critically what is taught and how it is being taught.

In evaluating different styles, it is helpful to learn about the origins, philosophy, and founder of the particular hatha yoga tradition you are interested in. There are fewer lineages than there are teachers, and by researching the master's approach (many of whom have written books on their teachings), you can obtain vital information about the aims and philosophies of different styles of hatha yoga. By examining the cultural roots of traditional yogic teachings, you can assess them in the light of your own values, needs, priorities, and experiences.

While all styles of hatha yoga are beneficial, some have specific physical requirements. To know which style is right for you, pay careful attention to how your body responds to the postures. If you haven't exercised in a while or have tight muscles (particularly hamstring and back muscles), relying on props to gain correct alignment may be necessary. This doesn't mean that you and this type of yoga are incompatible. Give yourself time to understand the poses and your body time to get acquainted with becoming flexible in unfamiliar areas. If you aren't sure if one style is better for you than another, give it a trial run of at least three weeks before deciding. To make a fair evaluation, take careful note of how you feel after a class. You should feel centered and calm, stretched but pushed beyond your limits. Over the long haul, yoga classes should have a positive effect on your well-being.

If you have any health concerns about your health or fitness, consult your physician, qualified health practitioner, or yoga teacher before undertaking a yoga practice, especially with these specific health problems: high blood pressure, heart disease, arthritis, back or neck injury, or recent surgery.

HOW TO FIND THE RIGHT TEACHER

Yoga classes and teachers vary tremendously. Each teacher instructs from his or her own experiences, thus furthering the tradition of direct transmission from teacher to student and the on-going evolution of yoga.

The American Yoga Association defines a good yoga teacher as one who:

- has spent time studying the various effects of yoga exercises, breathing, and meditation
- has a working knowledge of major muscle groups and body systems
- is able to vary techniques according to each person's individual capability
- will not confuse the yoga techniques by allowing his or her own religious beliefs to affect the class

Tips for Locating a Qualified Yoga Instructor

- Decide what you want to learn and at what pace.
- Ask a friend for a recommendation.
- Check the local Yellow Pages, YMCAs, local newspapers, health food store and church bulletin boards, and metaphysical bookstores for information about local instruction.

If there are no instructors in your area, contact teachers in nearby areas for recommendations. Also, the yoga associations listed in the Resources section of this book can refer you to instructors in your area.

Both *Yoga Journal* and *Yoga International* magazines produce annual directories of yoga teachers and studios located in the United States, Canada, and abroad. The *Yoga Journal* list is featured in the magazine's July/August issue and is also available by mail. The *Yoga International*, published in the January issue, list is available through its regular subscription service or by special order.

Before taking a class, call the teacher to discuss her or his style and emphasize and your needs or expectations. Ask about teaching experience and qualifications.

Determine if the class size is right and if classes are conducted in an organized fashion. Are the instructions clear? Is there individual attention and gentle correction, both verbal and hands-on?

After attending a class, ask yourself whether you find the style of teaching compatible.

Various yoga institutes, centers, ashrams, studios, and independent senior teachers offer training programs. Many of them also offer certification for aspiring yoga teachers who complete a specific course of study that stresses yogic philosophy, anatomy, postures, breathing techniques, meditation, and diet. However, programs vary in content and length of study and testing. Currently, yoga teachers are not licensed or certified by any national program and are exempt from regulation by individual states. However, this may change.

The *Yoga Sutras* suggest maintaining a relationship with one teacher. This relationship will help you reach a deeper understanding and greater degree of trust in him or her. In an atmosphere of trust, the teacher will be better able to discover what it is you need to learn. Following one teacher and one direction helps you discover ways and means to avoid and overcome the various obstacles that come up in practicing yoga.

HOW TO BE A GOOD YOGA STUDENT

Like everything else in life, yoga takes time to learn and understand. It also has its share of ups and downs. One day it may seem effortless, and the next it's a struggle to bend over and reach your toes. Like any exercise program, your yoga practice should consist of warm-up poses, work toward more challenging poses, and end with a cool-down and relaxation period.

Yoga can help us stay centered when times are good, bad, and in-between. Even when we think practicing is a waste of time and energy, it is not. When thoughts such as this arise, remember that the act of practice itself, sticking to our commitment, is valuable. Esther Myers, a long-time Canadian yoga teacher, explains that "yoga trains us to center and release…consistent practice takes commitment and discipline, tempered by compassion and self acceptance and finding the way that is right for you."

While yoga is calming and centering, it is also a vehicle for expressing and clearing strong energy and emotions, with specific poses to deal with the turmoil. While doing poses you like is important to sustaining and enjoying a solo practice, your routine should be well-rounded and should include some poses from all the major groupings of poses: standing, inversions, twists, forward bends, backbends. When beginning a yoga practice, emphasize standing postures, as they will strengthen major muscles quickly, thus providing a solid base for other postures.

Be enthusiastic. Initially, your eagerness for learning yoga may be high but may waver over time. A commitment to learning anything worthwhile requires patience and dedication, as well as renewing or reconnecting with the energy or reason for pursuing the study in the first place. Don't rely on your teachers to always pump up your enthusiasm to learn and practice.

Be open to learning from different teachers, but be careful not to take classes from too many different teachers at the same time. This also applies to attending workshops. Attending classes regularly or taking the occasional workshop is fine, but not at the expense of not developing or ignoring your own private practice. Take the time to integrate what you've learned from your teachers into your own practice before attempting more.

Be curious. Iyengar yoga expert Donna Farhi suggests one way to develop curiosity is to cultivate "disbelief" for the purpose of exploring and investigating on your own. Farhi encourages students to observe themselves carefully while in a posture. She suggests asking these questions: How does this movement affect my body? What happens if I do it another way? How am I reacting to this posture?

Without these elements, according to Farhi, there is no real learning. She urges students, regardless of where they are in their yoga practice, to regard yoga as an ongoing process rather than a single accomplishment.

Yoga can be a life-long pursuit, but persistency, consistency, and discipline are required to gain the many lasting benefits yoga offers. This news should encourage your effort and strengthen your resolve. There is no hurry, and the fear of loss should not concern you. The yogic scriptures state that no effort is lost or wasted on the path of knowledge.

Tips for Serious Yoga Students

• Be on time. This is important if you take yoga instruction seriously. Arriving ten to fifteen minutes early is advised so you can get into the proper frame of mind and warm up. Important instructions often are given at the beginning of class. Chronic lateness is a sign of disrespect to both the teacher and fellow students.

- If just starting or getting reacquainted with yoga, sign up for a beginner's class or practice only the basic postures and routines.
- Be attentive. You're apt to learn more and grasp complex ideas more readily. Put the events of the day aside while in class. Students who are motivated and interested inspire teachers to go out of their way to help them progress.
- Be seen. Introduce yourself to the teacher, preferably before the start of class. Don't hide in the back; position yourself near the front.
- Be consistent. Your progress and the quality of class are enhanced by regular attendance. Hatha yoga, like any skill, is gained through steady, mindful accumulation of knowledge and practice. This means going to class when you don't feel like it.
- Don't compare yourself with anyone else. Individuality extends to levels of flexibility as well as body types. While it is human nature to compare, remember, yoga is noncompetitive and we all learn at different rates.
- Go at your own pace, moving gradually into each pose.
- Listen to your body. Stretching is good, pain is not. Yoga does not "go for the burn."
- Set reasonable goals, taking into account your current physical condition, degree of flexibility, and age.
- Proceed slowly when trying new poses. The mind needs time to absorb the new movements and the body to get used to them.
- Keep mind and body relaxed. When your attention wanders, bring it back gently to the yoga.
- Be appreciative of constructive criticism. Verbal and hands-on correction are typical in many of the styles of hatha yoga. Take it in the manner it was intended—to help you along the path.
- Be appropriate when asking questions. Most teachers welcome students' questions during class, as both the class and teacher can learn from them. Questions should be brief and

pertain to the matter at hand. Questions not pertaining to the current subject or those of a personal nature should be asked after class.

- Be appreciative of your teacher. Offering encouragement or feedback when something a teacher does is helpful (or potentially harmful) can be a morale booster, as well as bettering the quality of his or her teaching.

- Don't give up. The initial discomfort or struggle with adapting your body to the postures eventually disappears and gives way to more positive feelings.

- The more you practice the more benefits you derive. You don't have to be an expert or master to feel and look better in a relatively short period of time.

THE IMPORTANCE OF A PERSONAL PRACTICE

If you are attending regular classes, you might ask yourself why it is important to develop your own personal practice—an excellent question. Developing a personal practice goes beyond the notion of taking time or caring for yourself.

Working alone and at your own pace leads to discoveries that may not come to light during class, when you are mainly following instructions. When practicing on your own, you can spend time working on problem areas, such as lower back, shoulders, and hamstrings, or becoming more familiar with basic postures before moving on to more challenging ones.

In addition, yoga masters have determined that two years of diligent practice is required before the student fully understands the nature of the poses and begins to appreciate how they are interconnected. Patañjali wrote that the mastery of *asanas* occurs only when practice becomes effortless.

How to Establish a Personal Practice

Set a goal—whether it is stress reduction, weight loss, increased flexibility, enhanced immunity, or heightened spiritual awareness—your motivation should be personal. Remember that it takes time to perfect the posture.

Set aside a regular time to practice, as yoga frees and relaxes the body to do other things. Practice regularly, even if it's only a few minutes every day. More time, however, will deepen your practice as well as your satisfaction with it. With regular practice, tight muscles will release, and as they do, poses will become easier to do. The amount of time and effort given to practice brings equivalent results.

It may take some experimenting to determine your optimal time of day and length of practice. Steady, regular practice will help you stick to your routine on days when you don't feel like it or don't see the progress you had hoped for. As your practice develops over time, the positive effects of yoga will appear more subtle and perhaps less noticeable.

If possible, establish a regular time of day to set aside for practice. Morning or evening practice is advised. Practice when your body is most limber. Some people find their bodies are stiff in the morning, making practice more difficult. Night practice, however, may limit the kinds of postures you do as some are too stimulating and affect sleep. Whatever schedule you devise, do it long enough to see how it works, including on weekends.

Practice at the same time each day for fifteen to twenty minutes. Add another five to ten minutes to your practice every three to four weeks. The key is regularity.

Start with your favorite poses. Repeat them two or three times before moving on to the next *asana*. While in the pose, do not hold the breath. Between postures, take one or two breaths to quiet the mind.

Be patient. Some people are genetically less flexible or have tighter muscle groups than others. But this doesn't mean real progress can't be made. Stretching overly tight hamstring and neck and shoulder muscles takes some getting used to. Conversely, overflexibility presents problems as well.

When beginning, practice every other day, up to four days a week. Gradually work up to six days of practice, and rest on the seventh. Enjoy whatever time you have set aside for practice. One experienced teacher put it quite well: "It's better to practice just a little and enjoy it than to not practice at all."

How to Prepare for Practice

Have an empty or near empty stomach. Wait a minimum of ninety minutes after eating before practicing postures and four hours after a large meal. If very hungry before class, eat some yogurt or fruit.

Wear comfortable clothing that keeps you warm, but not too warm—leotards, unitards, cotton tights, bike shorts, loose T-shirts or tank tops. Bulky or overly loose clothing will only get in the way. Practice barefoot to avoid slipping.

Set aside a special place to practice. If you use props (wooden blocks, belts, folding chair, etc.), store them together and set aside or bring to the practice area before beginning.

When indoors, set the thermostat to sixty-five to seventy-five degrees. Keep a blanket or sweatpants handy for Corpse or other complete relaxation poses and meditation. If practicing outdoors, select a shady spot with plenty of room to move. Dress accordingly.

For seated meditation, use firm blankets folded three or four times lengthwise or a firm pillow or cushion specifically made for meditation.

Minimize distractions. Turn off the radio, TV, and telephone, and set the answering machine volume to the low setting. Clear the room of pets and kids, if possible.

Locate a level surface. A bare hardwood floor is ideal, but if your feet slip, use a sticky mat. If practicing on carpet, choose an area with a tight weave, such as Berber.

How to Get the Most from Your Practice

The effects of practicing yoga are cumulative. If done every day or nearly every day, even ten to fifteen minutes will help build concentration, increase flexibility, and strengthen willpower, making it easier to practice the next day. Consistency is key. Most yoga instructors believe that there is more benefit to doing a brief practice regularly than hit–or–miss home practice sessions, sporadic class attendance, or the occasional workshop. Veteran Canadian yoga teacher Esther Myers says the value of an on-going practice cannot be over-estimated. As yoga germinates and takes root in your life, you will find the rhythm and level of practice that is right for you. The greatest and longest-lasting benefits are achieved when at least three or four yoga *asanas* are done every day.

When starting, realistically assess how much time you can devote to yoga practice. Then start with poses you find you can master easily and work toward more challenging ones.

Adjust your practice to your schedule and biorhythms. Some days will find you not feeling as energetic or flexible, even weak or tired. On those days, try doing restorative poses, such as supine poses and forward bends.

Don't practice when you have a fever. If you have a cold or other minor illness, use your judgment and restrict your practice to restorative ones.

Be aware that some poses affect mood and energy differently. Poses that are more stimulating include Sun Salutation, backbends, and standing poses. These poses are best done early in the day. More appropriate for the evening are forward bends, inversions, and restorative poses. Hero's Pose, Reclining Hero's Pose, Bound Angle Pose, and Basic Sitting Forward Bend are ideal for relaxing and recharging. Reclining Hero Pose is especially beneficial after consuming a heavy meal, as it aids digestion. (See the following chapter for directions for specific poses.)

One way to extend your yoga practice is to incorporate yoga throughout the day. In your daily routine, there are many ways you can practice yoga without actually doing a formal posture such as:

- Relax by exhaling and dropping your shoulders when standing or sitting. Repeat several times throughout the day.
- Straighten your spine when sitting, standing, and walking.
- Lift your chest while driving.
- Take several deep breaths that expand the diaphragm.
- When standing in line, spread your feet, straighten ankles; when walking, be conscious of touching the ground with entire surface of the foot.

How Long Should You Practice?

Most experts recommend a minimum of ten minutes of practice every day. However, to practice a range of postures and incorporate breathing or meditation, fifteen to twenty-five minutes is necessary. These brief practice sessions should also be interspersed with longer sessions of thirty to ninety minutes three or four times weekly.

To move forward in your practice, longer practice sessions of at least forty-five minutes to an hour are required. Extended practice sessions should include a specific breathing practice with a long relaxation period. However, you should never practice to the point of exhaustion. If you are overly tired or sore after a regular practice session, you may be too practicing too long or attempting postures that are too advanced or strenuous.

If you're new to yoga or if you've been sedentary or you spend long hours sitting in front of a computer screen, the muscles in your legs—hamstring and calves specifically—hips, shoulders, and lower back may be sore. After practice and before retiring, take a long hot bath spiked with a couple of cups of Epsom salt to reduce the stiffness you might experience the next day. Severe muscle or joint stiffness means you've overdone it and gone past your maximum. Give your body a chance to recover by resting and, if your body permits, very light stretching. However, if you have severe pain that doesn't lessen in twenty-four hours, muscle cramps, headaches, or dizziness or any other unusual symptoms, see your doctor.

Practicing During Menstruation and Pregnancy

Inverted postures, which turn the body upside-down, should be avoided while menstruating. Some methods suggest refraining from practicing yoga postures during the first forty-eight to seventy-two hours. However, when you feel discomfort, forward bends may be done in moderation.

During the early stages of pregnancy, inversions can be continued if you have practiced them before. If pressure or breathing problems occur at any time, come out of the pose immediately. Practice of *pranayama*, without holding the breath, is encouraged as a preparation for labor.

How to Practice

Pay attention to your body. Check your alignment from head to toe for balance and stability before beginning any posture. Feet should make firm contact with the ground with toes spread. Weight is evenly distributed. Ankles are firm and straight, not rolling in. Kneecaps are lifted. Hips and shoulders are level. Chest and stomach are lifted. Shoulders roll back and down. Collarbone spreads. Chin is level. Neck balances comfortably between the shoulders. Mouth and throat are relaxed.

Pay attention to the instructions, particularly the directions for placement, as they form the foundation of the pose. Strive for correct body alignment.

- For most postures, socks should be removed before beginning. Keep the eyes open in the postures except for Corpse Pose. Relax the facial muscles and keep the eyes soft.
- Move slowly into the pose to avoid injury and to more easily feel which muscles are actively working.
- Go as far into the pose as comfortable, to a point where you can maintain the pose in correct alignment, not necessarily to its maximum. Work on the edge of the stretch, but back off if there is any pain. Listen to how your body responds.
- Don't bounce, as this shortens rather than lengthens the muscle. Bouncing creates an automatic resistance and risks injury.
- Breathe. Slow down and take the time to focus your attention on your breathing. Breath should always be taken in through the nostrils and out through the mouth.

- Hold the pose as long as even breathing is maintained. Time will increase as the body becomes more familiar with the poses and strength and flexibility increase.
- Don't hold the breath while in a pose, as it tightens the body. Use the breath, particularly exhalation, to facilitate the stretch.
- Smile when you do a posture; it helps you relax and enjoy what you're doing.
- Turn attention inward. Pay attention to how your body feels—where it's tight, strong, or tired. Practicing *asanas* provides valuable feedback.
- Avoid tensing muscles around the eyes, jaws, neck, throat, shoulders, and stomach. Keep your eyes open in the poses, except in Corpse Pose.
- If a pose hurts, stop and rest. There is nothing in yoga that says no pain, no gain.
- Don't tense when encountering discomfort, as this further tenses the muscles. Be calm and gentle and remain open to releasing the blocked area. If in pain, come out of the pose, and adjust the pose or add a prop to reduce the amount of stretch.
- Pay attention to your body. Trust your body's response to being in a pose. It is ego that pushes the body past the point of endurance often causing harm. Never force or push yourself into a pose or hold a pose past the point of real endurance.

Learn to distinguish between discomfort and pain. Joint pain in the neck, knees, lower back, or hips should mean to release the posture and rest. Muscles that are tight, particularly the hamstrings and the ones surrounding the hips and shoulders, will take time to lengthen and relax. As you work these muscles, begin slowly, increasing their capacity to stretch over time.

When adjusting a pose, start from the ground up. In standing poses, begin with the feet; for inversions, start with the head, shoulders, and elbows; and in seated poses, begin with the sit bones and position of the pelvis.

Don't "muscle" your way into poses through strength alone. Instead, smile, breathe, and relax and lengthen the muscles you're working.

To end the pose, come out the same way as going into it. Focus on alignment, keeping the breath steady.

Rest for a minute after three or four consecutive poses, especially when practicing standing poses. Recommended "resting" *asanas* are Standing Forward Bend and Child's Pose.

During menstruation, do not practice Headstand, Shoulderstand, the intense standing poses (Side Angle Pose, Intense Side Stretch and Warrior I & II), or backbends, as they reverse the flow of blood.

If you are nursing an injury or have high blood pressure, are pregnant, recently injured, or have chronic back pain, consult with your doctor and a qualified yoga instructor before beginning a yoga practice.

How to Stay Motivated

In his wisdom, Patañjali identified eleven obstacles to yoga practice:

- lack of interest
- self-doubt
- laziness
- sensuality
- false knowledge
- failure to concentrate
- pain
- despair
- sickness

- unsteadiness of body
- unsteadiness of respiration

Interestingly, only four of these obstacles have to do with physical limitations; the rest are concerned with the mind, reflecting the connection between body, mind, and spirit.

Even the most advanced yoga students have had to overcome some limitations imposed by their bodies. Beginning students, especially, must keep their expectations realistic. Achieving lasting flexibility comes in small increments over long periods of time. Conversely, don't use unrealistic expectations as a reason not to practice or to quit altogether. Every posture has a beginning, middle, and advanced stage. Props will help you to accommodate physical limitation. Holding poses for only brief periods can offer as much benefit as holding them for longer periods.

Staying Motivated

Vary your sequence or add new postures. Continue to spend time in the more familiar poses even as you add new ones.

Create space in your home for yoga, even if it's only a corner of a room. It will reinforce your commitment to a regular practice. Besides props, you might include a small bookcase to store reference books and videotapes. Add photos, candles, or incense or put up a yoga calendar for atmosphere and inspiration.

- Wear a special outfit. It offers the psychological advantage of separating yourself from the other parts of your day.
- Experiment with interesting and unusual props. Props help achieve proper alignment in postures. Try sofas, doorways, or stairs, in addition to the regular yoga props (blankets, bolsters, wood blocks, belts, etc.) Always use caution when trying a pose with a new prop.

- Find a friend to practice with and set a date and time for practice. Even if your buddy fails to show, practice anyway.

- Remind yourself why you do yoga. Don't you look and feel better—calmer, stronger, more flexible, balanced, poised—since you started practicing yoga?

- Study yoga; it's inspiring. Your local library probably has a wealth of books and videos on the subject.

- Make yoga a priority. Assigning a high priority to yoga will strengthen your commitment to regular practice. Commitment helps push through habitual procrastination and avoidance behavior. If you're a chronic procrastinator or have an extra-busy schedule, schedule time in your calendar for yoga practice. Making a date takes the hassle out of finding the time; with time scheduled in, there's no debate.

Basic Postures for Health and Relaxation

OVERVIEW

Yoga postures, or *asanas*, are the physical positions that coordinate breath with movement and with holding the position to stretch and strengthen different parts of the body. *Asana* practice is the ideal complement to other forms of exercise, especially running, cycling, and strength training, as the postures systematically work all the major muscle groups, including the back, neck, and shoulders; deep abdominal, hip, and buttocks muscles; and even ankles, feet, wrists, and hands.

By their very nature, *asanas* affect major and minor muscle groups and organs as they simultaneously impart strength, increase flexibility, and bring nourishment to internal organs. Although most poses are not aerobic in nature, they do in fact send oxygen to the cells in the body by way of conscious deep breathing and sustained stretching and contraction of different muscle groups.

CATEGORIES OF ASANAS

There are a wide variety of *asanas* (up to 200), each one with its own distinct shape and form dictated by stretches, counterstretches, and resistance. The result is an alignment of the skin, flesh, and muscular structure of the body with the skeleton. When done with conscious breathing, the postures balance the sympathetic and parasympathetic nervous systems. These two major parts of the nervous system govern the automatic functioning of the internal organs, heart rate, blood pressure, automatic breathing, and digestion.

Yoga postures and sequences offer many benefits. For instance, forward bends, twists and inversions stimulate the entire internal system, including the lymphatic system, and boost the immune system. Other poses stimulate, calm, and energize, while others build stamina or concentration, promote sleep, alleviate PMS, or soothe digestion.

Asanas are grouped by their main physical characteristic, and each group of postures develops the body in a different yet reciprocal way. *Asanas* also are characterized by the three basic movements, including backbends, forward bends, and twisting movements.

What the Poses Represent

Through practice of the *asanas*, you learn how to sit or stand erect, stable, and relaxed without being tense and rigid or collapsing and falling asleep. One great master of therapeutic yoga declares: You should do all *asanas* with vigor and at the same time be relaxed and composed.

- standing poses = vitality
- sitting poses = calmness
- supine poses = restful
- prone poses = energizing
- backbends = liveliness
- inversions = mental strength
- twisting poses = cleansing
- balance poses = lightness
- jumpings = agility

See Appendix for illustrations of poses described in this section.

Standing Poses

These poses invigorate the mind and body by eliminating tension, aches, and pains. Internally, these postures stimulate digestion, regulate the kidneys, and alleviate constipation, as well as improve circulation and breathing, by developing the strength of the legs and the flexibility of the pelvis and lower back. Through regular practice, standing poses lend strength and mobility to the hips, knees, necks, and shoulders.

Standing poses are important for beginning students, as they teach the basic principles of alignment and movement in sitting, standing, and walking. In addition, they establish a firm foundation for learning other postures. Standing poses are recommended for daily practice for students of all levels because they exert a tremendous effect on the neck, shoulders, legs, and back.

Standing postures include:
- Mountain Pose (*Tadasana*)
- Tree Pose (*Vrksasana*)
- Triangle Pose (*Trikonasana*)
- Standing Forward Bend Pose (*Uttanasana*)
- Wide-spread Standing Pose (*Prasarita Padottanasana*)
- Side Angle Pose (*Parsvakonasana*)
- Warrior I & II (*Virabhadrasana I & II*)
- Intense Side Stretch Pose (*Parsvottanasana*)
- Half Moon Pose (*Ardha Chandrasana*)
- Revolved Triangle Pose (*Parivrtta Trikonasana*)

Standing poses are typically begun by jumping into them, which makes the body and mind alert and develops coordination. In jumping, the feet should land equidistant from the center and in line, and the arms should move out to the sides at the same time with the legs. People who have back or knee injuries and pregnant women should not jump into standing poses, but walk the feet outward to the sides to begin the pose. For support and to better gauge alignment, these poses can be practiced against the wall.

Caution: Standing poses should not be practiced during the first few days of menstruation, the first three months of pregnancy, or by anyone with a problem pregnancy or high blood pressure or heart problems.

Sitting Poses

Generally, these poses are considered calming, as they soothe the nerves, eliminate fatigue, and refresh the brain. They also help regulate blood pressure and assist in recuperation from illness, as well as promote restful sleep. Sitting poses are divided into two categories: upright seated postures, which involve bending the legs into different positions, and forward bends, where the trunk bends over the legs.

The primary sitting postures include:

- Staff Pose (*Dandasana*)
- Hero Pose (*Virasana*)
- Lotus Pose (*Padmasana*)
- Cow's Head Pose (*Gomukhasana*)
- Bound Angle Pose (*Baddha Konasana*)

Forward Bends

Also known as seated postures, these poses stretch the lower back and lengthen the hamstrings. They are considered passive poses that encourage introspection and cool the internal body. Specifically, sitting forward bend postures soothe the nervous system and quiet the mind. They can be approached two ways—either energetically, with a vigorous breath, or calmly, with a quiet breath. When practiced with the forehead resting on a bolster or stack of folded blankets and held for several minutes, these poses are restorative, and they are especially recommended during menstruation. They are useful after a series of backbends as they serve as a counterbalance to the body.

Forward bends postures include:

- Open Angle Pose (*Upavista Konasana*)
- Head-to-knee Pose (*Janu Sirsasana*)
- Revolving Head-to-knee Pose (*Parivrtta Janu Sirsasana*)
- Seated Forward Bend Pose (*Pascimottanasana*)
- Seated Forward Bend (with one leg in Hero Pose) Pose (*Triang Mukhaikapada Pascimottanasana*)
- Tortoise Pose (*Kurmasana*)
- Heron Pose (*Krauncasana*)

Reclining Postures

These poses fall into two categories—supine and prone poses. The prone poses rejuvenate the body. Reclining poses serve mainly to stretch the abdomen and increase the mobility of the spine and hips, thus opening the groin and strengthening the back, arms, and legs.

The less strenuous of these poses traditionally are done at the end of a practice session to cool down the body and restore energy. The postures also are helpful for relieving fatigue, recovering from illness, or during menstruation. When used as a restorative series, the eyes frequently are covered and props such as folded blankets, bolsters, and belts are used to facilitate their remedial effects. When supported with props such as folded blankets or bolsters, these poses can be held for five to ten minutes each.

Reclining postures include:

- Legs Up the Wall Pose (*Viparita Karani*)
- Reclining Head-to-foot Pose (*Supta Padangusthasana*)

- Reclining Hero Pose (*Supta Virasana*)
- Reclining Bound Angle Pose (*Supta Baddha Konasana*)
- Corpse Pose (*Savasana*)

Backbends

Backbends open and energize the body and mind; they develop courage, energize, and lift depression. They open the chest, stimulate the nervous system, strengthen the arms and shoulders, and increase flexibility of the spine. Since these poses are strenuous, they should be introduced gradually to a steady yoga practice. To avoid risking injury to the lower back, the legs first must be strong, and the shoulders and upper back must exhibit genuine flexibility. Backbends should not be done by those who have high blood pressure, heart disease, or other serious illness, or during menstruation and pregnancy. Those with bad backs or knee injuries should only do backbends under the supervision of a qualified yoga instructor.

Backbend postures include:

- Bridge Pose (*Setu Bandha*)
- Bow Pose (*Dhanurasana*)
- Camel Pose (*Ustrasana*)
- Upward Facing Dog (*Urdhva Mukha Svanasana*)
- Upward Bow Pose (*Urdhva Dhanurasana*)

Inverted Poses

Along with arm balances, inverted poses reverse gravity, bringing fresh blood to the head and heart, thus revitalizing the whole body. These poses tone the internal organs and glandular system, stimulate brain function, improve circulation, and refresh tired legs.

In particular, Shoulderstand invigorates the nervous system and regulates the emotions while activating the thyroid. To avoid straining the neck, this pose should be done with the shoulders and elbows supported by two or three firm, folded blankets, which can be staggered slightly for neck comfort. Headstand is considered the "king" of yoga postures, as it fosters poise and stimulates the brain. New students should practice Downward Facing Dog as a preparation before attempting Headstand.

Inverted postures include:

- Downward Facing Dog Pose (*Adho Mukha Svanasana*)
- Handstand (*Adho Mukha Vriksasana*)
- Headstand (*Salamba Sirsasana*)
- Shoulderstand (*Sarvangasana*)
- Elbow Balance (*Pinca Mayurasana*)
- Plow Pose (*Halasana*)
- Supported Bridge Pose (*Setu Bandha Savangasana*)

Caution: These postures should not be done during menstruation or pregnancy, or by anyone who has high blood pressure, migraine headaches, heart problems, detached retina, glaucoma, neck problems, ear problems, or hiatal hernia. Those with neck injuries should do these poses only under the direction of a qualified instructor.

Twists

These postures free, energize, and balance the body. Sitting twists are the most intensive, as they increase the range of motion of the spine. They promote flexibility in the spine, hips, and upper back, thus relieving backaches, headaches, and stiffness in the neck and shoulders. This group of postures also tones and stimulates the abdominal organs, thus aiding digestion and relieving constipation.

Ideally, twisting postures are done after a series of sitting poses or forward bends, which gives the hips and spine a proper warm-up. When done after backbends, they tend to relieve any lower back discomfort. They should not be done during pregnancy, with the exception of the Chair Twist (*Bharadvajasana*).

Twisting postures include:

- Seated Twist Pose (*Maricyasana*)
- Simple Chair Twist Pose (*Bharadvajasana*)
- Severe Twist Pose (*Ardha Matsyendrasana*)

Balance Poses

Balance poses develop lightness, strength, and agility. They also help develop body control, muscle tone, coordination, and concentration. These poses are not recommended during menstruation or pregnancy or after recent (twelve to eighteen months) abdominal surgery.

Balance poses include:

- Plank Pose (*Chaturanga Dandasana*)
- Sideways Plank Pose (*Vasisthana*)
- Crane Pose (*Bakasana*)

Practice Suggestion

Remove contact lenses when practicing reclining poses (when eyes are covered) or doing inversions.

BASIC CLASSIC YOGA POSTURES

After Headstand, the Lotus Pose is most familiar to Westerners. *Padmasana*, as it's known in Sanskrit, requires long and limber muscles in and around the deep ball-and-socket that make up the hip joint. Initially, this pose may be nearly impossible to accomplish, due mostly to sitting in chairs for long periods of time, which leads to the muscles and ligaments around the hip joints becoming short and tight.

Attempting this pose in its complete form without proper preparation and warm-up can result in injury, especially to the knees, because when the hips are tight there is a tendency to overstretch the knees. Lotus Pose should never be forced under any circumstances. It takes patience and practice to master. All the standing poses are excellent preparation, as are Easy Pose and Tailor's Stretch, described below.

Easy Pose (*Sukhasana*)

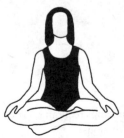

Sit on the front edge of a firm, folded blanket with legs crossed. Knees should be parallel to the floor with your weight balanced evenly on the sit bones. Move shoulders down, lift crown of head until chin is level. Hands should rest comfortably on knees. Breathe in and out slowly and deliberately. (If knees are four to six inches off the ground, support with pillows or wooden blocks.)

Tailor's Stretch

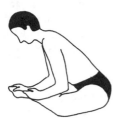

Start in a relaxed cross-legged position. Begin moving the feet away from the groin until legs form right angles. Now hold this position and move the spine forward until an intense stretch is felt in the outside of the hip. Change the crossing of the legs and repeat.

Lotus Pose (*Padmasana*)

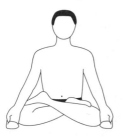

Sit in Easy Pose. Then take the right foot with the heel and bottom of foot pointing toward groin and place on the left thigh. Right hip should roll in with knee facing almost forward. Then raise left foot forward and upward and place on right thigh. Feet should move closer toward groin; move knees closer together. Straighten back, lift chest. Rest hands with palms facing up on the top side of knees. Be careful not to strain knees. Hold for ten to thirty seconds, breathing evenly.

Mountain Pose (*Tadasana*)

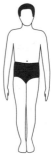

The foundation for all hatha yoga postures, this pose centers and calms the mind and teaches balance.
Stand straight with head centered over the legs. Bring feet together with big toes and ankles touching. Weight should be balanced evenly on both feet and toes should be elongated and

not gripping. Lift the arches. Legs should extend fully, lifting the kneecaps and pulling the thigh muscles up and inward toward the bones. Then lift the hips, while moving the lower back down, tucking the pelvis under. Without tensing the stomach muscles, move them up and back. Arms should hang loosely at your sides. Raise the breastbone and relax the shoulders and flatten the shoulder blades. Stretch the neck upward and keep the head straight and chin level. Relax facial muscles, especially the muscles around the eyes. Look straight ahead. Hold for thirty to sixty seconds.

Downward Facing Dog (Ahdo Mukha Svanasana)

This pose, like many others, has a few variations. It provides an excellent method for stretching the shoulders and hamstrings and helps relieve depression, insomnia, and stress. This variation is for beginners.

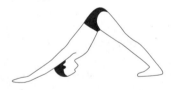

With back to wall, kneel on all fours. Then place hands shoulder-width apart and six inches ahead of shoulder level. Position knees directly under the hips with heels on the wall and ball of foot on the wall. Spread toes fully. Then exhale and raise trunk, straighten knees, and move buttocks upward toward ceiling. Hold position with toes and balls of the feet spread fully. Keep head lowered. Slowly bring heels down wall and continue to spread the toes and balls of feet. To come out of the pose, return to kneeling position. Hold for thirty to ninety seconds.

Legs Up the Wall Pose (*Viparita Karani*)

An excellent posture for relieving stress and refreshing the body, this pose also invigorates the legs and feet.

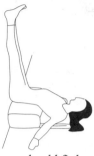

Place the long side of two double-folded blankets or a bolster parallel and about six to ten inches from the wall. Then sit at one end of the prop, facing away from it, with one shoulder near the wall and hips close to the wall. Roll toward the center of your prop, bring your legs up and parallel to the wall. The ribs closest to your waist should be supported by the bolster. Your abdominal area now should fit between the end of the bolster and the wall. Remember to maintain a curve in your neck, supporting your neck with a thin blanket or towel if necessary. Rest your arms either beside you on the floor or over your head with elbows bent. To come out, bend your knees and place your feet on the wall. Lift your pelvis slightly away from the prop. Push the prop toward the wall with your hands and press your feet against the wall to bring your body away from the wall. Then rest the lower part of your legs on the bolster and lie there for a few moments. Then roll to your right side and get up slowly.

Child's Pose (*Pranatasana*)

This relaxation is often done between asanas or asana sequences.

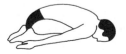

Start with knees on the floor. Place hands on the floor in front of knees. Then sit back, resting on the back of the calves. Hands now rest lightly on knees. Then extend hips and hands forward. Let palms rest on floor. Relax shoulders. Head can be turned so either the left or right cheek rests on the floor. Forehead can also rest on the floor. Relax in the position, inhaling and exhaling several times before coming out.

Sun Salutation (*Surya Namaskar*)
This pose invigorates the entire body with stretches and counter-stretches.
The classic sequence yoga posture, Salute to the Sun features several hatha yoga poses done in a continuous fashion. Depending on how it is performed, the posture can be mildly to very aerobic. Ideally, the pose is done in the morning. Movement should be synchronized with breathing and should be done twice in each set, alternating between leading with the left and right foot. This variation is for beginners.

First, stand in Mountain Pose and stretch the arms overhead, palms together, bending slightly backwards. Then bend forward from the hips, resting your hands on your shins, ankles, or toes, wherever your flexibility permits. If necessary, bend your knees slightly to eventually bring palms flat on the floor beside your feet. Extend the left leg back, with the knee resting on the floor. Right knee should remain at a ninety-degree angle before bringing the right foot back to join the left foot. Then lift the hips toward the ceiling to form Downward Facing Dog, with arms straight, back long and head facing downward. If necessary, move hands back a bit to lift hips. Or move hands and feet to a wider stance. Bend the arms at the elbow, then lower hips and place knees on the floor, followed by the trunk. With arms bent, extend the body in a straight line behind you.

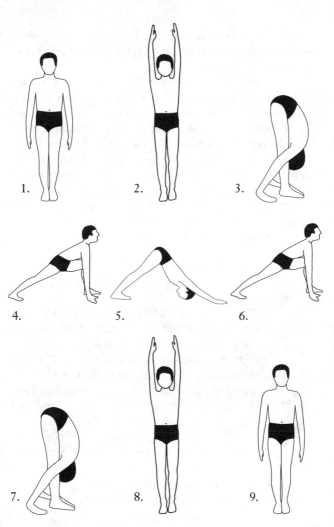

Stretch should be in lower back. Use arms to bring chest area forward; relax shoulders. Eyes look forward. Navel should be off the floor.

Now lift hips again and reposition hands until you are in Downward Facing Dog. Then bring the left foot forward between the hands. If necessary, drop the right knee and lift the foot with the opposite hand to bring it forward. Then bring the right foot forward. Both legs should be straight. If this strains your lower back, bend knees slightly. Hands should rest on shins, ankles, or toes, head moving toward the legs. With arms at your side, roll trunk up slowly. Once upright, bring arms over head with palms together and bend slightly backwards. Release and bring hands to a prayer position at the breastbone.

Headstand (Salamba Sirsasana)

This classic posture activates the brain and develops equilibrium and inner strength.

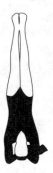

To practice, start in Child's Pose. Move forearms out until elbows are on the floor at the width of the shoulders. Hands can be resting on the floor or fingers interlaced and hands clasped. Wrists should be resting firmly on floor. Lengthen the spine with shoulders moving downward to floor. Shift weight until you are balancing on hands and knees. Bring head between hands with crown (top) of head resting squarely on floor. Keep hands and fingers active yet relaxed. Extend the back of the neck.

To advance in the pose, straighten legs as in Downward Facing Dog Pose, lift hips toward ceiling while standing on your toes, then gradually move heels toward floor. Walk feet in toward head.

When you are ready to do the full pose, place a firm, folded blanket against a plain wall. Kneel in front of the blanket; knees and feet should line up. Interlock the fingers and move them to the edge of the blanket, facing the wall. Forearms and outer elbows should also be on the wall, with elbows under the shoulders. Forearms, wrists, and hands are parallel. Cup hands and extend the neck, placing the very top, or crown, of the head between hands. Lift upper arms and shoulders. Lift and straighten legs and elevate the hips. Walk legs toward wall until nearly perpendicular. Then swing either the left or right leg upward so it is parallel to the wall. Lift shoulders and stretch the back of neck. Stretch legs and trunk; tuck lower back inward. Feet, heels, and toes extend upward. Face and eyes should be relaxed with a soft focus. To release, extend one leg toward the floor, then bring down other leg. Rest in Child's Pose.

Bridge Pose (*Setu Bandha*)
A simple backbend, this pose opens the chest, helps to deepen breathing, and strengthens the lower back.

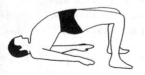

Lie on your back on the floor with knees bent and feet hip-distance apart. Feet should be close to the buttocks. Extend arms toward heels with palms down. Waist rests lightly on floor with feet pressing down firmly. Tuck chin slightly. Lengthen spine and lift pelvis off floor until weight is evenly distributed between shoulders and feet. Keep knees steady at hip distance. Lengthen spine again, breathe deeply. To come out, exhale and roll spine down to floor. To release lower back, clasp hands around knees and rock gently back and forth.

Corpse Pose (*Savasana*)

This posture, which represents stillness and quietness, balances the nervous system. It typically is done at the end of a practice session.

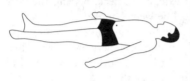

Keep two blankets handy—one to support the neck and the other to cover the front of the body should you become chilly.

Sit on the floor with the trunk upright. Lean back on the elbows with the head moving downward, trunk and legs in a straight line. Rest on the center of the back of the skull. Stretch neck and throat. Relax the eyes. Chin should be level. If it is higher than the forehead, place a blanket folded to a one to two inch height under the head until it touches the top of the shoulders. Shoulders move down with shoulder blades moving in. Then bend knees, lift up hips, and stretch lower back toward floor. Straighten legs and let them roll comfortably outward. Relax and extend arms about six inches from the trunk. Wrist and hands also rest on floor. Relax the abdomen. Close eyes and focus attention on the in and out breath. Let body sink into floor. Remain in pose for five to ten minutes.

To come out, open eyes slowly, bend the left leg and roll to your right side, remaining there for a few breaths. Use left hand to slowly bring you to an upright position.

SEQUENCING

Moving from one pose to another without breaking form is called "sequencing," or *vinyasa* in Sanskrit. This method of practice allows for a balanced workout regardless of practice length.

Sequences can consist of related poses for the purpose of energizing (as with standing poses or backbends) or relaxing (with forward bends or restorative poses) the body or working on specific areas such as the hips, shoulders, or feet.

Whatever the purpose of a particular practice session, it should begin with two or three warm-up postures, such as Mountain Pose, Downward Facing Dog Pose, or Sun Salutation, as they stretch the spine, arms, and legs. Then you can move on to more strenuous poses that strengthen the body and increase endurance. Standing, inverted, and backbend poses would apply here. To wind down and settle the nerves, practice seated forward bends or supine poses. Always end with several minutes in Corpse Pose to renew both mind and body.

MINIMUM PRACTICE GUIDELINES

According to Iyengar yoga teacher, Esther Myers, the ideal minimum practice should consist of:

- Supported Inverted Pose (*Viparita Karani*)
- Downward Facing Dog Pose (*Adho Mukha Vrksasana*)
- Triangle Pose (*Trikonasana*)
- Bridge Pose (*Setu Bandha*)
- Headstand (*Salamba Sirsasana*)
- another Downward Facing Dog
- Child's Pose (*Pranatasana*)

(See *Starting a Hatha Yoga Practice* for important information and tips about performing yoga poses.)

PROPS

Some schools of hatha yoga rely heavily on props, while others do not. If you are new to yoga, have limited flexibility, are practicing mainly on your own, or are taking a therapeutic approach to yoga practice, including props is quite appropriate.

The most commonly used hatha yoga props include:

- Yoga ("sticky") mat: offers a nonslippery surface for standing postures

- Two or three tightly woven or firm blankets: Woolen army-type or Mexican blankets are ideal. Used in sitting poses when there is tightness in the hips or hamstrings, for support in Shoulderstand, Headstand, and Corpse Pose.

- Two wooden or dense foam blocks (approximately 4 in. x 6 in. x 9 in.) for support in standing poses and Hero Pose (*Virasana*) and Elbow Balance Pose (*Pinca Mayurasana*).

- Belt with a buckle for Bound Angle Pose, forward bends and Shoulderstand.

- Folding chair with a flat seat for supported backbends and standing and twisting poses.

Pranayama: Working with the Breath

Prana is the breath of life of all beings of the universe.

—B. K. S. Iyengar

YOGIC BREATHING

As a yogic practice, *pranayama* concerns itself with various methods of conscious breathing. *Prana*, or vital force, is at the core of all life. All living beings are infused with it; without this form of energy, life could not exist. Eastern religions have long recognized that training the breath is important to mental, physical, and spiritual growth. However, many people are shallow chest-breathers, taking in only about one-third of the oxygen needed by the lungs. Chest breathing is closely linked to the workings of the nervous system. By gaining control over diaphragmatic breathing, you greatly enhance your ability to cope with stress and lessen its damaging effects. Yogic breathing emphasizes breathing through the nose and the exhalation over the inhalation.

The classic text on yogic breathing, *Light on Pranayama* (Crossroad Publishing, 1987) by B. K. S. Iyengar, instructs that the conscious breathing system of *pranayama* provides a direct avenue of communication to the self. Iyengar says that the practice of *pranayama* quickly induces the relaxation response and accompanying enhancement of the immune system.

The *Yoga Sutras* declare that the more balanced and calm we are, the less *prana* is lost to us. When we are restless, upset, or befuddled, more *prana* exists outside the body than within, potentially leading to physical illness. When there is too little *prana* for the body to draw upon, we can feel stuck or less motivated to do what needs doing. Distinguished teacher Desikachar states: "If *prana* does not find sufficient room in the body there can only be one reason: It is being forced out by something that really does not belong there. When we practice *pranayama*, it is nothing more than reducing the 'rubbish' and so concentrate more and more prana within the body...the quality of our breath influences our state of mind and vice versa because we can influence the flow of *prana* through our breath. In yoga we are trying to make use of these connections so that *prana* concentrates and can freely flow within us."

CONNECTION TO HATHA YOGA

Hatha yoga strives to bring the body into balance, and *pranayama* lends stability to the body's energies. Yoga postures involve the most basic *pranayama* practice: paying attention to the breath. By practicing yoga *asanas*, we have the opportunity to become aware of our breathing and to affect it in some way. Yoga tests, or challenges, the way we breathe. The postures give us a new perspective on the muscles used in breathing, as they require you to twist, bend, and invert our bodies. Paying attention to the breath becomes important because for the pose to be done correctly both breath and movement must be coordinated. As a result, the connection between mind and breath is strengthened. Yoga poses automatically increase lung capacity and invigorate the muscles most directly involved in the breathing process—specifically the ribs, diaphragm, and back.

As yoga postures strengthen the body for meditation, *pranayama*, while much more subtle a practice, prepares the mind for the silence and single-pointed concentration required of meditation. A steady and correct hatha yoga practice naturally encourages the practice of *pranayama*.

Resting poses offer the most opportunity to become more aware of the muscles involved in the breathing process. They include:

- Corpse Pose (*Savasana*)
- Easy Pose (*Sukhasana*)
- Lotus Pose (*Padmasana*)

UNDERSTANDING INHALATION AND EXHALATION

Both an involuntary and voluntary action, breathing is the act of moving air in and out of the lungs. Inhalation brings oxygen, and, therefore, energy into the body. Exhalation removes impurities from the body and creates the space for *prana* to enter the body. The out–breath is considered key because it removes any obstacles to the free flow of *prana*.

However, bringing *prana*, which is not simply air or breath, into the body involves something more. Yogic scholars believe *prana* enters the body when a positive change in the mind occurs over an extended length of time. Desikachar noted that "changes of mind can be observed primarily in our relationships with other people." He further reminds that relationships are the real test of whether we actually understand ourselves better.

FORMS OF PRANAYAMA

There are five forms of *prana*, all of which have different names according to the body functions with which they correspond. The forms most Westerners practice are *prana-vayu* and *apana-vayu*. *Vaya* means "air" or "breath" in Sanskrit.

- *udana-vayu*—corresponds to the throat region and the function of speech
- *prana-vayu*—corresponds to the chest region
- *samana-vayu*—corresponds to the central region of the body and the function of digestion
- *apana-vayu*—corresponds to the region of the lower abdomen and the function of elimination
- *vyana-vayu*—corresponds to the distribution of energy into all areas of the body

BENEFITS

Like *asana* practice, *pranayama* practice has far-reaching, positive effects on physical, emotional, and mental well-being. It also encourages spiritual development. More specifically, mindful breathing practice:

- clears and calms the mind
- focuses attention
- develops concentration
- refreshes and renews the body
- improves metabolic function
- assists in cardiovascular function

BASIC METHOD

Working with the breath takes time, patience, and concentration. Initial attempts at *pranayama* may be frustrating. You may find the process absorbing yet distracting at the same time. Before attempting any particular technique, breathe normally, without trying to control or change your breathing in any way. Practice this way until you are comfortable in letting your breath–flow freely. Lying down (as in the Corpse Pose or with the knees bent, feet flat on the floor) on a firm surface instead of sitting upright in a classic meditation pose may be helpful as you experiment in becoming familiar with your breathing pattern.

As you become quieter, your breath will find its own rhythm and will naturally become steadier and slower. Inhalation and exhalation will become fuller and deeper on their own. As your flexibility grows through *asana* practice, so will your capacity to deepen the fullness of your breath. Practicing *pranayama* may require a leap of faith, but through practice and patience you can master it.

Ideally, *pranayama* should follow *asana* practice, and not the other way around. At least ten to twenty minutes of rest should occur between the end of *asana* and the start of *pranayama*. Finding the ideal sitting position for *pranayama* practice also is important. Comfort is essential, so you can remain in a seated position for an extended period of time while keeping the spine straight. Most practitioners opt for Easy Pose or a variation of the Lotus Pose, either with or without back support from a wall. If your hips are tight, elevate them by sitting on a folded, firm blanket. Hands can rest in your lap or rest lightly on the knees.

In the *Yoga Sutras*, Patañjali offers these suggestions for keeping your attention on or conscious of the breath:

- Focus on a place in the body where you can feel or hear the breath; this is most easily achieved by gently contracting the vocal cords, a technique known as *ujjayi*.
- Follow the movement in the breath, feeling the inhalation from the center of the collarbone, down through the rib cage to the diaphragm, and following the exhale upward from the abdomen.
- Pay attention to the breath where it enters and leaves the body at the nostrils.
- Also helpful is softening the eyebrows, broadening the forehead, relaxing the eyes so that they recede, resting back in their sockets.

Should you experience any of the following signs of stress or tension as you practice *pranayama*, stop the technique immediately and resume regular, passive breathing:

- tension in the chest, neck, or shoulders
- strain in the foreheads, eyes, or throat
- a forced sound in the throat when breathing
- gasping for the inhalation
- lightheadedness or hyperventilation
- feeling tense, overstimulated, or lightheaded afterward
- more emotional release than feels comfortable

How to Breathe

- Keep mouth closed and take in breath only through the nose.
- Keep your breath slow and smooth and focus your attention inward. Pay attention to the sound of your breath. It should be steady and even.
- To even out the flow of the breath, try making a very slight, quiet sound at the back of your throat.
- Inhale and exhale should flow consistently. Avoid bringing in or expelling breathe loudly or forcefully.
- Pause slightly between inhalations and exhalations.
- Do not strain or force any part of this process. Give yourself the chance to find a rhythm that is comfortable for you. Remember that the breath is connected directly to your nervous system and regulating the breath manipulates both gross and subtle energies. Shallow or agitated breathing signals a stress response.

Breath Retention

The breath should be held or retained when breathing in and out fully can be accomplished with ease. The purpose of retaining the breath during *pranayama* is to quiet the mind. Retaining the breath should not interfere or disturb the inhalation-exhalation pattern. If the exhalation becomes rough or uneven, resume regular breathing.

Breathing Techniques

Pranayama includes many techniques that are based on the Complete Yoga Breath, which includes the chest, diaphragm, and belly moved by the breath. Techniques such as *Ujjayi*, *Viloma*, and Alternate Nostril Breathing should be practiced only when the breath can be regulated with ease—ideally, when an *asana* practice has been established. Those with breathing problems such as asthma or chronic shortness of breath should practice under the supervision of a trained teacher. When practicing any form of *pranayama*, you must remain mindful of how the body reacts during the process.

Basic Techniques
Reclining

Lying down is an ideal way to practice when beginning or if you are tired or ill. The spine is automatically supported; by resting in a prone position, you can relax more readily.

1. Begin in Corpse Pose. Support the head with a firmly folded blanket if there is strain in the neck or the chin is higher than the forehead.

2. Pay attention to the flow of your breath. Make no attempt to adjust or control your breathing. Inhale and exhale passively. Inhaling slowly, place one hand lightly on the abdomen. As you inhale, feel the abdomen expand and contract when you exhale.

3. After several cycles of inhalation and exhalation, allow the entire body to sink closer to the floor and deepen the exhalation.

Sitting

Sitting upright and comfortable is the ideal posture for *pranayama*, as it frees the upper body and aids in concentration.

1. Sit in a cross-legged position. Back and hips may be supported; if knees are higher than the hips, sit on a firmly folded blanket high enough that spine is straight and knees are lower than the hips. Spine may be supported by sitting against the wall.
2. Lengthen spine and soften the abdomen. Lift breastbone and relax the arms and shoulders. Lower back is neutral. Head rests comfortably on the base of the spine and chin points downward. Soften eyes, eyebrows, and forehead.
3. Facial muscles, eyes, and gaze remain passive. Jaw is relaxed.
4. Inhale and exhale normally, observing the breath's natural rhythm.

Extended Exhalation

This technique helps take breathing to the next level by deepening exhalation and increasing the volume of inhalation.

1. Breathe normally while paying attention to the movement of the abdomen.
2. When breath becomes rhythmic, slowly bring the muscles of the abdomen toward the spine as you exhale.
3. Let the knees and pelvis move downward as the spine and upper body move upward.
4. Keep inhalation passive as you continue the cycle.

Square Breath

This technique is very effective for steadying the breath and subsequently calming the mind. It calls for pausing briefly at the end of each inhalation and each exhalation.

1. Breathe normally until breath is steady and rhythmic.
2. Pause after the in–breathe and again after the out–breath.
3. Slowly increase the length of the pauses until the inhalation, the exhalation, and the two pauses that are part of the cycle are the same length.

Meditation

OVERVIEW

The subtlest parts of yoga's Eight-fold Path are:

- *pratyahara*—withdrawal of the senses from the physical world
- *dharama*—concentration
- *dhyana*—meditation
- *samadhi*—union with the Higher Self

Taken together, these elements represent what Westerners commonly call meditation, a natural progression from the more physical aspects of yoga practice. At its most basic, meditation is considered an effective, albeit low-tech, antidote to stress and an unfettered path to mindfulness. In the broadest sense, however, meditation can be characterized as a focusing of attention. It is very much part of the Eastern tradition, as Indian philosophy and medicine made its way to Tibet, China, Japan, and Southeast Asia. How it was taught and practiced was altered by the cultures that absorbed it.

While the object of attention may vary, all forms of meditation have as their goal the centering of one's attention, or mental energies, for the purpose of stilling the mind. A very reliable way to calm an overactive mind, meditation also increases physical stamina, mental concentration, and spiritual resolve. Regular meditation practice instills a sense of living in the present moment—facing pleasant and unpleasant emotions, thought patterns, fears, and cravings without distraction.

BENEFITS

Like the other yogic paths, meditation is nondenominational and offers many potential benefits to both mind and body, including:

- stress relief
- peace of mind
- relaxation
- increased energy
- release of tension
- lower blood pressure
- mindfulness
- access to higher mindstates

METHODS

There are many ways to practice meditation. The most basic and easiest mediation style to learn is to simply sit straight and quiet with eyes closed and concentrate on the breath—inhalation, then exhalation, then inhalation again, and exhalation—while not engaging the thoughts that pass through the mind. Some practices extend the observation of the breath to observing the sensations, thoughts, and emotions of the mind and body. When attention wanders, as it invariably will, meditators are instructed to gently bring their attention back to their breathing. Forcing the mind to be still only results in frustration.

Choosing a meditation method is much like adopting a form of hatha yoga or selecting a teacher. It depends greatly on what strikes a chord within and how compatible it is with your lifestyle. It is an important decision and should be made with care and consideration. Instead of accumulating techniques, stick with one style until you've mastered it.

Regardless of the method chosen, meditation requires patience, understanding, and practice. As with learning and perfecting yoga postures, meditation is a lifelong quest.

Corpse Pose (*Savasana*)

Hatha yoga students are most often introduced to meditation through Corpse Pose, which is done at the conclusion of each practice session. This pose brings about deep relaxation, as the body is still, yet passively alert and fully supported by the floor. In the pose, muscles relax and lengthen, passive breathing—necessary in all postures—takes over, and quiet concentration builds (see also page 74).

Postures

The traditional postures for sitting meditation include:

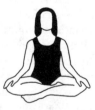

• Easy Pose (*Sukhasana*)

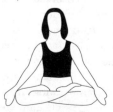

• Accomplished Pose (*Siddhasana*)

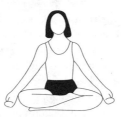

• Auspicious Pose (*Swastikasana*)

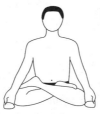

• Lotus Pose (*Padmasana*)

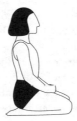

• Thunderbolt Pose (*Vajrasana*) for Buddhist and Zen meditators
• Sitting upright in a straight chair, if you are unable to sit in a crossed-leg posture.

Whichever pose you choose, you should be able to sit comfortably with the spine and head erect, allowing for the free flow of energy throughout the body. The body should remain still and relaxed, with the mind aware yet internally focused. Sitting on a firm cushion or folded blankets supports the hips and relieves lower–back strain.

The hand position can be either resting loosely clasped in the lap; hands cupped but open, with the right hand on top of the left, resting lightly on the lap; or the thumb and forefinger touching and the hands placed on the knees.

While not encouraged, beginning meditators may find it easier to quiet the mind and follow the breath when lying on the floor in Corpse Pose. If you find yourself becoming drowsy or falling asleep, try meditating this way at a different time of the day.

ESTABLISHING A PRACTICE

Deciding when, where, and how long to practice comes first. A regular time and place, while ideal, is not mandatory.

According to Indian gurus, the best time to meditate is between 4 A.M. and 6 A.M. This time of morning is known as *brahamuhurta*, the time when the mind is infused with peacefulness and goodness and stillness exists in the outside world, as many people are still asleep. Other recommended times are 6 A.M., noon, 6 P.M., and midnight.

A quiet place free of clutter, distractions, and interruptions is essential for meditation. If this place can be set aside only for meditation, all the better. In fostering a spiritual atmosphere, you may want to set up a small shrine that holds candles, fresh flowers, sacred objects, photos of inspirational spiritual masters, and other objects of personal importance. The room should be neither too cold nor too warm; fresh air should circulate to help keep you alert while meditating.

The best way to start a meditation practice is to sit for daily for five or ten minutes. After the habit has been established, gradually lengthen the amount of meditation time in five-minute increments. If you become tense or very restless, reduce the time by five minutes. You may find after a few weeks that as you meditate more, you look forward to the time you've set aside. However, should you want to expand meditation to more than an hour each day, it is best to do this in a group setting or under the supervision of a qualified teacher.

To free the body from tension, repeat the ancient mantra *Om* several times; as it is believed to represent the fundamental sound of the cosmos, the vibrations will dispel areas of tension.

Traditional Yogic
Diet Principles

OVERVIEW

The ancients have known all along what science and health practitioners are rediscovering today: diet plays a significant role in sustaining and restoring good health and well-being and maintaining a smooth–functioning nervous system. Today, research continues to support a plant-based diet—one that is low in fat and rich in complex carbohydrates—to prevent and treat heart disease; some types of cancer; digestion disorders, including gallbladder disease; diabetes; and hypoglycemia. Such a diet also allows for others to eat well and helps ensure the health and continuation of planet Earth.

The yoga of food is called *anna* yoga. According to yogic scriptures, food can affect us in three ways: it provides nourishment for energy, strength, and emotional equilibrium; it can be the source of illness and mental confusion; it can impede function, which leads to sickness and even death.

The yogic ideal encourages cultivation of the *sattavic* foods in the diet to encourage a state of mind that is lucid, alert, and capable of higher realizations. The most revered of the yogic scriptures, the *Bhagavad Gita*, offers specific dietary advice on how certain foods will cultivate a particular nature. While yogic scripture contains much dietary advice, the overriding guiding principles in a yogic diet are to eat minimally and to fast regularly.

FOOD CATEGORIES

Yogic philosophy divides foods into three categories—*tamasic*, *rajasic*, and *sattavic*. It recommends avoiding tamasic and rajasic foods as they can upset physical, mental, and emotional equilibrium. *Sattavic* foods, on the other hand, encourage energy, clarity, and creativity.

Tamasic Foods
- stale, over- or under-ripe foods
- meat, fish, mushrooms, and vinegar
- frozen and canned foods
- overcooked and reheated foods
- drugs and alcohol

Rajasic Foods
- sour, bitter, and acidic foods
- coffee, tea, onions, garlic, and eggs
- chocolate, white sugar, and flour
- strong spices and hot peppers

Sattavic Foods
- fresh fruits and vegetables
- milk, butter, beans, and honey
- cereals
- fresh fruit juices
- pure water

In more modern times, the traditional yogic diet has been decidedly lacto-vegetarian, including dairy products with the exception of eggs. Eating eggs has largely been discouraged, as they possess a *rajasic*, or stimulating, quality while bean and grain combinations and soy food are favored, as they provide protein and do not cause negative effects on the mind and body. Milk and related products possess *sattavic* nature; dairy foods are reputed to be easily digested, easy on the system. However, milk is considered a food and should be consumed slowly.

VEGETARIANISM

The basic principles of the yogic diet are good health and common sense and hence, vegetarianism. This type of diet is thought to encourage compassion for all living things, a more refined mind, and a higher consciousness. Certain foods help the mind to become more refined, and others keep it at the consciousness level of an animal.

The basic yogic diet features:

- vegetables and herbs
- fruits
- nuts and seeds
- grains
- legumes
- specific dairy products such as yogurt and ghee (clarified butter)

Ideally, these foods are consumed raw or lightly cooked to preserve their life force or *prana*.

However, the decision to become a partial or total vegetarian should not be forced. It should be undertaken willingly and only if there is no risk to maintaining health. Not everyone is cut out to be a vegetarian. Your body may require the nutrients found only in meats or in more concentrated quantities. On the advice of his doctors, even the Dalai Lama does not practice vegetarianism, although many of his followers do. To a yogi, however, health reasons are secondary to the idea of nonviolence. The concept of nonviolence includes not only refraining from harming living creatures, but also from harming oneself. To start out on the road to vegetarianism by forcing yourself to eat differently before you are ready or doing it because you think you should is a form of violence. Eliminate meat from your diet gradually, and explore other sources of protein.

There are several types of vegetarian diets:

- lacto-ovo, where dairy products and eggs are permitted
- lacto-vegetarian, which allows dairy products but no eggs
- vegan, which refrains from dairy products
- fruitarian, where only "fallen fruits"—so no plants have been destroyed during harvesting—are consumed
- macrobiotic diet, similar to vegan but with a heavy emphasis on consuming brown rice

A regular hatha yoga practice helps us become more aware of our eating habits and reduces cravings for junk food. As a result, many practitioners find it easier to maintain a healthy weight.

HOW TO EAT HEALTHFULLY

During her many trips to India, its adopted daughter and revered yoga teacher Indra Devi acquired dietary advice that she has passed on to her students over the years:

- Do not overeat.
- Avoid dead foods—ones that have been robbed of their natural vitamins, minerals, amino acids, and enzymes by processing. This includes canned, preserved, pickled, bottled, bleached, polished, and refined foods.
- Eat plenty of fresh fruits, salads, and vegetables or fruit and vegetable juices every day.
- Drink lots of fresh water.

- Inhale a sufficient of quantity of fresh air.
- Eat foods that support the "rate of life," or metabolism. The best foods include vegetables, particularly the green variety, fruits, whole grains, honey, oils, nuts, milk, eggs, fish, and meat. These foods contain all the necessary vitamins, minerals, amino acids, and enzymes, the life-chemicals that control metabolism.

Serious yogis also avoid consuming alcohol, as it is in direct opposition to yoga's purpose. Alcohol lowers the vibrations of the astral body, while the purpose of yoga is to elevate these vibrations. Eating meat is also thought to have a detrimental effect on the astral body.

WATER

Most of us don't drink enough water. By the time thirst sets in, so has mild dehydration. Eight-tenths of the body consists of water, and we eliminate about two quarts every day—even more in higher altitudes. Insufficient water intake is responsible for constipation, a congested colon, malfunction of the liver and kidneys, and clogged bowels. As a general rule of thumb, drink one glass of water each day for every fourteen pounds of body weight. For most of us, this translates to five to eight glasses of water daily.

As a rule, yogis never drink cold water or water with ice. This is particularly important during meals, as it impairs the flow and potency of the enzymes necessary for digestion. Ideally, water should be consumed at room temperature. A glass of fresh, pure water is recommended first thing in the morning and last thing at night. If constipated, drink water hot with some lemon. On hot days, try hot water or herb tea with honey or lemon, as it actually cools the body.

FASTING

In the yogic context, fasting goes beyond skipping meals or starving oneself as a form of discipline. Fasting, when done for spiritual and health purposes, should be approached with the same seriousness and dedication as practicing *asanas*, *pranayama*, or meditation.

Benefits of Fasting
- removes toxins and poisons from the body
- rejuvenates *prana*, or life energy
- purifies the mind
- furthers spiritual practice
- expedites the removal of waste materials from the bowels, kidneys, skin, and lungs
- engenders a feeling of lightness and freshness
- rests the digestive system

How to Fast

Fasting monthly for a period of twenty-four hours is considered the most practical and efficient method for busy Westerners. However, fasting is not appropriate for people with these health conditions: diabetes, kidney disease, bulimia, or anorexia. It is also not advised for those who have recently undergone a detox program for drug or alcohol dependency.

Drink only mineral water or diluted fruit juice and nothing else. Drink plenty of water. If fasting more than two days, use a small amount of fresh lemon juice. Lemon juice is a natural disinfectant for the stomach and cleanses the liver and kidneys.

Rest as much as possible, doing light yoga stretches, restorative poses, *pranayama*, meditation, and walking outdoors.

Eat lightly upon breaking the fast, slowly introducing solid foods.

TONGUE AND NOSE CLEANING

Both these hygiene customs have been long practiced in India and Nepal, using special equipment to accomplish the task. A curved, stainless instrument is used to scrape away the coating of impurities that build up over time on the tongue. This cleaning is best done in the morning before drinking or eating to avoid washing the collected impurities into the digestive system. A spoon, used in an inverted position, can do the job nicely.

Irrigating and cleansing the nasal passages is done with a *neti* pot, a small ceramic pot with a bowl and spout for mixing the right amount of warm water with a pinch of salt. Besides aiding breathing, running water through the nose also helps to keep the sinus passages healthy.

Appendix

STANDING POSES

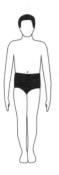

Mountain Pose
(*Tadasana*)

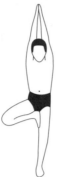

Tree Pose
(*Vrksasana*)

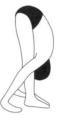

Standing Forward
Bend Pose
(*Uttanasana*)

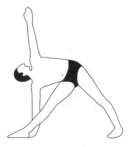

Triangle Pose
(*Trikonasana*)

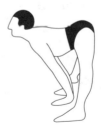

Wide-spread Standing Pose
(*Prasarita Padottanasana*)

STANDING POSES (cont.)

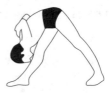

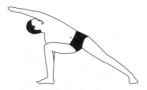

Side Angle Pose
(*Parsvakonasana*)

Intense Side Stretch
(*Parsvottanasana*)

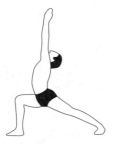

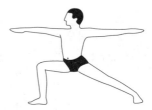

Warrior I
(*Virabhadrasana I*)

Warrior II
(*Virabhadrasana II*)

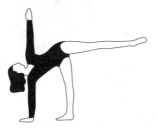

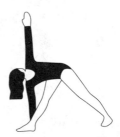

Half Moon Pose
(*Ardha Chandrasana*)

Revolved Triangle Pose
(*Parivrtta Trikonasana*)

SITTING POSES

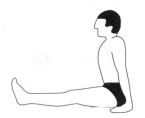

Staff Pose
(*Dandasana*)

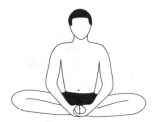

Bound Angle Pose
(*Baddha Konasana*)

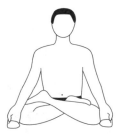

Lotus Pose
(*Padmasana*)

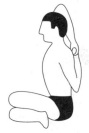

Cow's Head Pose
(*Gomukhasana*)

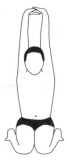

Hero Pose
(*Virasana*)

FORWARD BENDS

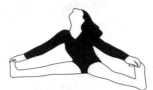

Open Angle Pose
(*Upavista Konasana*)

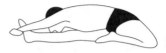

Head-to-knee Pose
(*Janu Sirsasana*)

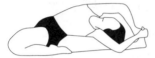

Revolving Head-to-knee Pose
(*Parivrtta Janu Sirsasana*)

Seated Forward Bend
Pose (*Pascimottanasana*)

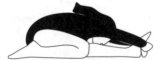

Seated Forward Bend
(with one leg in Hero Pose) Pose
(*Triang Mukhaikapada Pascimottanasana*)

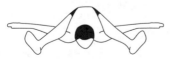

Tortoise Pose (*Kurmasana*)

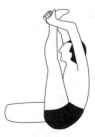

Heron Pose
(*Krauncasana*)

RECLINING POSTURES

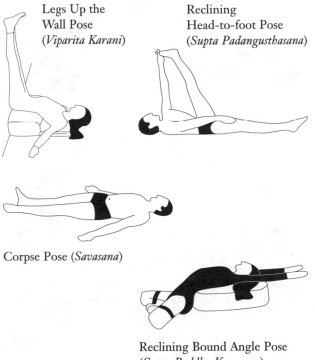

Legs Up the
Wall Pose
(*Viparita Karani*)

Reclining
Head-to-foot Pose
(*Supta Padangusthasana*)

Corpse Pose (*Savasana*)

Reclining Bound Angle Pose
(*Supta Baddha Konasana*)

Reclining Hero Pose (*Supta Virasana*)

BACKBENDS

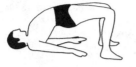

Bridge Pose (*Setu Bandha*)

Bow Pose (*Dhanurasana*)

Upward Facing Dog
(*Urdhva Mukha Svanasana*)

Upward Bow Pose
(*Urdhva Dhanurasana*)

INVERTED POSES

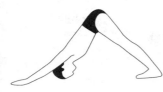

Downward Facing Dog Pose
(*Adho Mukha Svanasana*)

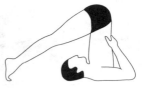

Plow Pose (*Halasana*)

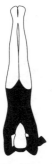

Handstand
(*Adho Mukha
Vriksasana*)

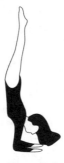

Headstand
(*Salamba
Sirsasana*)

Elbow Balance
(*Pinca Mayurasana*)

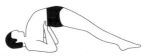

Supported Bridge Pose
(*Setu Bandha Savangasana*)

Shoulderstand
(*Sarvangasana*)

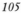

TWISTS

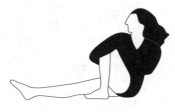

Seated Twist Pose
(*Maricyasana*)

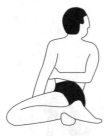

Simple Chair Twist
Pose (*Bharadvajasana*)

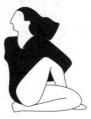

Severe Twist Pose
(*Ardha Matsyendrasana*)

BALANCE POSES

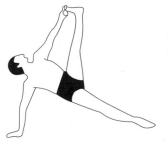

Plank Pose
(*Chaturanga Dandasana*)

Sideways Plank Pose
(*Vasisthana*)

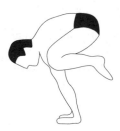

Crane Pose
(*Bakasana*)

Glossary

Asana—refers to all hatha yoga postures.

Bhagavad Gita—*Song of God*, classic yoga scripture of eighteen chapters; part of the epic poem, *The Mahabharata*. It describes the conversation between the warrior Arjuna and his spiritual advisor Krishna before a war. The story illustrates the need to find the necessary skills and courage to live life.

Easy Breath—an unconstrained but conscious breath pattern that is used when holding a yogic pose.

Eight-fold or Eight-limbed Path—the paths of yoga as decribed by Patañjali in the Yoga Sutras.

Hatha Yoga—the practice of yoga postures; word comes from *ha*, which means sun and *tha*, meaning moon. Yoga, taken from the word *yug*, means to yoke or to join and concentrate one's attention on.

Mantra—a particular word or phrase repeated mostly during meditation practice designed to evoke mindfulness.

Meditation—a deliberate state of withdrawal, conductcd in silence, where thoughts are suspended and the active mind is directed toward concentration on the breath, mantra, or specific subject, such as love, anger, or emptiness.

Om—serves as the root of all mantras and is the most well-known and popular of the mantras used to represent silence and stillness of the mind.

Namasté—traditional Indian greeting that acknowledges the existence of the other's innate goodness and godliness.

Patañjali—a sixth-century Indian who collected and systemized all the known knowledge of yoga and organized it into the *Yoga Sutras*. This written work is considered to be the "bible" of yoga, as it describes the purpose and methods of yoga.

Prana—represents the universal life force.

Pranayama—yogic breathing practice, which regulates and harmonizes the breath and its rhythm.

Pratyahara—contemplation or absorption.

Sutras—Sanskrit for the word "threads."

Yoga—means "mystical" and involves the union of the self with the Higher Self.

Yoga Sutras—Patañjali's classic text containing aphorisms on the meaning and practice of yoga.

Yogi—refers to any person who develops and maintains a committed yoga practice. In the strictest sense, it refers to one who has attained full realization of the self. A male practictioner of yoga is called a *yogin* and the female counterpart is known as a *yogini*.

Resources

American Yoga Association
513 South Orange Ave.
Sarasota, FL 34236
941-953-5859
Fax: 941-953-5959

Ananda Yoga
The Expanding Light
14618 Tyle Foote Rd.
Nevada City, CA 95959
800-346-5350
916-478-7518
Fax: 916-478-7519

Ashtanga Yoga/Power Yoga
325 E. 41st St., #203
New York, NY 10017
212-661-2895

B. K. S. Iyengar Yoga National Association of the United States
P.O. Box 941
Lemont, PA 16851
800-889-9642

International Association of Yoga Therapists
20 Sunnyside Ave., Suite A-243
Mill Valley, CA 94941
415-868-1147

International Kundalini Yoga Teachers Association
Route 2, Box 4 Shady Lane
Espanola, NM 87532
505-753-0423
Fax: 505-753-5982

Iyengar Yoga Institute of San Francisco
2404 27th Ave.
San Francisco, CA 94116
415-753-0909
http://www.iyoga.com/iyisf

Kripalu Center for Yoga and Health
P.O. Box 793, West St.
Lenox, MA 01240
800-741-7353
413-448-3152
Fax: 413-448-3384

Phoenix Rising Yoga Therapy Training
P.O. Box 819
Housatonic, MA 01236
800-288-9642

Sivananda Yoga Vendanta Center
243 W. 24th St.
New York, NY 10011
800-783-9642
212-255-4560
Fax: 212-727-7392

Viniyoga/T. K. V. Desikachar
The Pierce Program
1164 N. Highland Ave., NE
Atlanta, GA 30306
404-875-7110

**Yoga College of
India/Bikram Choudhury**
8800 Wilshire Blvd., 2nd floor
Beverly Hills, CA 90211
310-854-5800
Fax: 310-854-6200

Magazines
Yoga Journal
2054 University Ave., Suite 600
Berkeley, CA 94704
800-I-DO-YOGA
Fax: 510-644-3101
www.yogajournal.com
Also publishes an annual directory of yoga teachers in the U.S. and Canada.

Subscriptions:
Yoga Journal
P.O. Box 12008
Berkeley, CA 94712-9909
800-600-YOGA

Yoga International
RR 1 Box 407
Honesdale, PA 18431
800-821-YOGA
Also publishes an annual listing of yoga teachers regionally, nationally, and internationally.

Internet
The Yoga Finder
www.chesco.com/yoga finder
Web page for locating classes and teachers in the United States.

Videos
Living Arts
P.O. Box 2939
Venice, CA 90291-2939
800-254-8464
Fax: 800-582-6872

Pocket Guides from The Crossing Press

*Pocket Guide to Acupressure
  Points for Women*
ISBN 0-89594-879-6

Pocket Guide to Aromatherapy
ISBN 0-89594-815-X

Pocket Guide to Astrology
ISBN 0-89594-820-6

*Pocket Guide to Ayurvedic
  Healing*
ISBN 0-89594-764-1

*Pocket Guide to Bach Flower
  Essences*
ISBN 0-89594-865-6

*Pocket Guide to Celtic
  Spirituality*
ISBN 0-89594-907-5

Pocket Guide to Fortunetelling
ISBN 0-89594-875-3

Pocket Guide to Good Food
ISBN 0-89594-747-1

Pocket Herbal Reference Guide
ISBN 0-89594-568-1

Pocket Guide to Macrobiotics
ISBN 0-89594-848-6

Pocket Guide to Meditation
ISBN 0-89594-886-9

*Pocket Guide to Midwifery
  Care*
ISBN 0-89594-855-9

*Pocket Guide to Naturopathic
  Medicine*
ISBN 0-89594-821-4

Pocket Guide to Numerology
ISBN 0-89594-826-5

Pocket Guide to Self Hypnosis
ISBN 0-89594-824-9824-9

Pocket Guide to Shamanism
ISBN 0-89594-845-1

Pocket Guide to the Tarot
ISBN 0-89594-822-2

Pocket Guide to The 12 Steps
ISBN 0-89594-864-8

Pocket Guide to Visualization
ISBN 0-89594-885-0

Pocket Guide to Wicca
ISBN 0-89594-904-0